T0218626

A Handbook for Support Workers in Health and Social Care

Support workers are key deliverers of care in the UK, often hugely valued by those people they provide care for. Their roles and responsibilities are increasing in the midst of ever-changing health and social care systems. *A Handbook for Support Workers in Health and Social Care* recognises the contribution of support workers and provides an introduction to the core knowledge, legislation and models of practice required to work across health and social care settings.

Covering core person-centred skills that a support worker needs to develop, this textbook looks at knowing and managing yourself, before moving on to understanding your role in the organisation and teamwork. It outlines the relevant legislation and policies, from the Care Act (2014) to confidentiality. Communication, both written and in person, is a central theme, and key values such as compassion and dignity are explored in relation to this. There is a thought-provoking discussion of working with people, covering topics including respecting choices, thinking about risk and safeguarding. The book ends by looking at what it means to be a competent practitioner and the importance of continual professional development.

The first textbook introducing the core theory and practice knowledge necessary to work as a support worker in health and social care, it includes case studies, tasks and exercises to help the reader apply their learning.

The authors share more than 20 years of experience in the design and delivery of support worker courses in higher education. They deliver continuing professional development, bespoke training and consultation to the health and social care workforce.

Paul Mackreth is Course Director and Fellow of the Higher Education Academy in Nursing and Healthcare at Leeds Beckett University. Paul continues to maintain his nurse registration as a district nurse and is an active member of the Association of District Nurse Educators (ADNE).

Bryony Walker is Course Director and a Senior Fellow of the Higher Education Academy in Psychological Therapies and Mental Health at Leeds Beckett University. Bryony continues to maintain her registration as an occupational therapist and is a qualified coach working with health and social care managers.

A Handbook for Support Workers in Health and Social Care

A Person-Centred Approach

Paul Mackreth and Bryony Walker

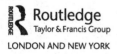
Routledge
Taylor & Francis Group

LONDON AND NEW YORK

First published 2021
by Routledge
2 Park Square, Milton Park, Abingdon, Oxon OX14 4RN

and by Routledge
52 Vanderbilt Avenue, New York, NY 10017

Routledge is an imprint of the Taylor & Francis Group, an informa business

British Library Cataloguing in Publication Data
A catalogue record for this book is available from the British Library

Library of Congress Cataloging-in-Publication Data
Names: Mackreth, Paul, author.
Title: A handbook for support workers in health and social care : a person-centred approach / Paul Mackreth and Bryony Walker.
Description: Abingdon, Oxon ; New York, NY : Routledge, 2021. | Includes bibliographical references and index. | Identifiers: LCCN 2020034664 (print) | LCCN 2020034665 (ebook) | ISBN 9781138036796 (hbk) | ISBN 9781138036802 (pbk) | ISBN 9781315178301 (ebk)
Subjects: LCSH: Allied health personnel–Great Britain. | Social service–Great Britain.
Classification: LCC R697.A4 M335 2021 (print) | LCC R697.A4 (ebook) | DDC 610.73/70690941–dc23
LC record available at https://lccn.loc.gov/2020034664
LC ebook record available at https://lccn.loc.gov/2020034665

ISBN: 978-1-138-03679-6 (hbk)
ISBN: 978-1-138-03680-2 (pbk)
ISBN: 978-1-315-17830-1 (ebk)

Typeset in Bembo
by Taylor & Francis Books

To my awesome daughter, Morgan. To my mum, Carol, for the unconditional love and support, and my late father, Colin, who would have been so proud, but would probably have never bothered reading the book. Finally, to Kitty Ricco for being an excellent friend through good times and bad times.

Bryony Walker

I would like to thank Joanne for her ongoing love and support; Tom, Sam and Luke ('the boys') for putting up with a grumpy dad; my parents and family for teaching me how to 'treat others as I would like to be treated', which I have used to develop skills in being empathetic; and my work colleagues for accepting and laughing at my cursing in front of the computer.

Paul Mackreth

To you, the reader.

We have written much of this book during two significant events with global impact: the coronavirus pandemic and the killing of George Floyd in the United States of America. We cannot express enough our gratitude and thanks to all those support workers, now understood to be key workers, who have given so much during the pandemic. Before the pandemic, we felt that you were undervalued in the workforce. The pandemic has shown how much you are needed and what you have contributed to health and social care.

The killing of George Floyd and other people of colour has shown us yet again that we have to call out 'Black Lives Matter'. How many times do we need to learn this lesson at the expense of people of colour? The role of support worker is probably one of the most diverse roles in health and social care. We should not have to write these words, but your lives matter.

Please accept this book as our gift to you, to help us all understand how valuable you are.

Contents

9   Know how to develop for new opportunities   92
BRYONY WALKER

Figures

Tables

Boxes

1 Introduction

Thank you for choosing to read our handbook. We anticipate that you have either done so because you are considering entering the field of practice called 'support work', or you have done so because you are already working in this field of practice and would like to learn more about it. We have written this handbook to provide you, a support worker in health and social care, with a core text similar to those that already exist for registered health and social care professionals such as nurses.

We have known for many years how important your role is in the delivery of health and social care. The Covid-19 pandemic has further shone a light on the important work that you deliver and, regrettably, how often it is still not appreciated or understood. If there is one thing that the Covid-19 pandemic has shown the public, it is that you are needed, valued by clients and families and have skills that you can develop further.

This handbook will provide you with a foundational understanding of and introduction to current core principles and values, legislation and models of practice required to work with the general public in a variety of health and social care settings. It will set the scene for a changing role (in the UK) where there are both opportunities and challenges in your support work practice. We, the authors – Paul Mackreth and Bryony Walker – are educators/academics involved in the design, delivery and evaluation of support worker courses in higher education. We have struggled to find an appropriate core text that captures, in a single publication, some of the generic knowledge necessary for support workers to understand their role. However, in the ever-changing world of health and social care, there are many recent developments for you and your colleagues to embrace, such as a code of conduct and the expectation that new support workers will have obtained a 'care certificate'. We found this lack of textbooks unusual, especially in the wake of policy-led developments and the publication of the historic Francis Report and the Cavendish Review, which both raised awareness that, like other health and social care practitioners, support workers must have access to training and educational opportunities. Both Sir Robert Francis (QC) and Camilla Cavendish understood, from their findings, that vulnerable people require care from support workers with a high level of competence and professionalism in their work.

To date, if you are interested in reading about the core skills needed for your role as a support worker or you just want to learn more to improve the quality of the care you offer, you have limited publications to view. You might have to look at the literature or research published for the registered professional workforce, such as registered nursing or therapy professionals. The authors encourage you to carry on doing this as a continuing professional development activity, but we also understand the importance of reading literature that relates to your professional identity, especially when there are an estimated 1.3 million support workers in the United Kingdom.

The title 'support worker'

In this book, we are attempting to start a conversation, make an assertion, that, although the support worker title is used generically, the role should be respected as a single discipline in its own right, as there is, across the sectors of both health and social care where you work, an overlap of knowledge, duties and responsibilities. The other professions are afforded this understanding.

How to read and use this handbook

We have attempted to make this book as accessible as possible and, where the chapters cannot provide all the necessary information, we request you engage in information-searching activity. We want to explore some of the 'norms' of practice to ensure that care delivery is exemplary and person-centred. As we will explore, this is often about getting the basics done well and getting it right the first time around.

In writing this book, we have walked the line of balancing giving information and allowing you time to consider the application to your own support work practice through small 'activities', which will be presented in boxes. We urge you to undertake these activities so that you give yourself time to think about your own practice.

This book is in handbook format so that you can consider making changes that improve your practice. Each chapter will follow the same style of giving you an introduction and some objectives (new things you will learn), setting the scene as to why each chapter topic is important, discussing areas within the topic (with activities) and then concluding what you will have learned. This is a common approach to most professional learning, and so you may want to get used to the process so that the handbook will set you up for your future study.

The chapters are presented in a logical order, moving from considering yourself, your clients and the context in which care takes place to aspects of that care support work practice. It concludes with recommendations for your future practice and continuing professional development (which some call life-long learning). We recommend that you start with Chapter 2 and work all the way through, in order, to Chapter 9. Don't do it all in one go. Perhaps read a chapter a week and work through it in 6–8 weeks.

We do recognise that many people don't read textbooks in this way. People often pick up a textbook, read the index page and then jump to chapters that they feel are interesting or relevant to their practice or an essay that they may be writing at that time. To this end, we have tried to make sure that each chapter can be read as a single topic in its own right. Each will link to other areas of the handbook, but can just be read as a single area of learning, so that you can dip into each chapter as a particular topic that you would like to read.

We hope that you enjoy reading it, but we cannot emphasise enough that reading is just the starting point. Take time to understand each topic. Link it to your practice area through the activities and, above all, keep on reading about those areas that most interest you through following up on some of the recommended other reading. Take time out to do this; you work in a busy, fast-paced practice environment and so you owe it to yourself and your clients to take time to read about how to practice.

Important themes throughout the handbook

Before you read the handbook, there are a few themes of 'practice' that are helpful to understand. We hope you have either observed or experienced them. Can you relate to them either in your role or in your journey to become a support worker?

The caring relationship

The most important message of this handbook concerns the person who requires your care and support. You may call them a client, patient or service user in your health and social care setting. We will use these terms interchangeably to reflect the different language across the sectors. We aim for you to be constantly aware of the person and their family (sometimes referred to as carers) as being at the centre of all that you do. We want you to put yourself in their shoes, even when the demands of your role distract you from this privilege. We have designed this handbook to be interactive to help raise personal and professional awareness that we hope will build your capacity for empathy and compassion and provide you with self-awareness to notice the warning signs that create barriers in the caring and supportive relationship.

Increasing roles and responsibilities of support workers

We frequently refer to 'context' in this handbook; this is everything in your practice that has an impact upon who you support and care for and how you fulfil your responsibilities. You will see in Chapter 3 that the support worker role is expanding; this is because of the workforce challenges such as skills gaps that are endemic across health and social care – gaps traditionally filled by the health and social care professional. However, it is also because clients' needs have changed to the extent that people need a lot of care and support for longer. We pose some questions for you to consider, ensuring that you can practise to the best of your ability and know where to get help and when to stop when an aspect of care or support falls outside your role.

Changing times: change in health/social care as a constant

Change is the only certainty in health and social care. The chapters in this book are, therefore, presented in a format that will allow you to search for your own reading material, both now and in the future. As authors, we cannot predict the future, but we can predict the future will look very different. What we intend to do in this book and in each chapter is to provide overarching principles and values that remain constant to ensure you put the client at the centre of your practice. So, although it is guaranteed that government health and social care policy will change and that what is good care and support will change, the overarching principle of keeping a client at the centre of care will not.

The need for an adaptable and flexible workforce to build career opportunities

In today's society it is unusual for any of us to have a job for life, for countless reasons, and we know from experience in the field that this is the same for the support worker. Support workers move posts to gain experience and broaden their career. Some people go into a support worker role as a stepping-stone to other things, taking promotional opportunities in leadership and management or training in one of the many health and social care professions. In Chapter 9, we aim to provide you with the knowledge to think about the future, whether you stay in your current position or would like to move on.

Being safe

One of the most important reasons for us writing this handbook and for you reading it is to improve the care and support that clients receive in health and social care. Each chapter of this handbook challenges the norms of practice and continually asks you if what you are doing is in the interest of your client. We all want clients to receive safe and effective care, but does this mean best care? There are always things that we can do differently and sometimes better. We need to continually improve the quality of practice. Through doing this, we can be assured that clients are safe and also that your practice is safe and competent and you are self-aware to avoid habits that are detrimental to delivering good care and support to vulnerable people.

Valued as the key deliverers of care by clients and family

Finally, and in conclusion, we intend to convey to you within this handbook that you are valued as a support worker, by your clients and their families. As you grow in your professional and personal awareness, your value to them will continue to grow and get stronger. You are in the unique position of offering time to your clients and focusing on the relationship. Across the sector, support worker responsibilities might range from carrying out intimate basic care needs to supporting the person to achieve a lifetime ambition; in some roles, you become a core part of the trusted family network. Your clients are watching you and assessing you, noticing your attention to detail in the care and support you offer.

2 Knowing yourself

Bryony Walker

Introduction

This chapter focuses on the importance of you, the health and social care support worker, being active in your efforts to understand yourself, as a human being, within your own relationships with family, friends and your wider social circle. Self-awareness can provide you with a lot of information that is meaningful for working in the care sector and can help you improve relationships and achieve goals in your own personal and professional life. We argue that, if you hope to have a long-term career in the field of health and social care, aside from studying and training within the field, you will need to work hard to understand yourself in order to do the best for the patients, service users and clients you work with. The chapter will provide you with some activities to engage in and some models and tools that are sometimes used in health and social care training, but are also used other sectors such as counselling, business and commerce to build self-knowledge and self-awareness.

Learning outcomes

At the end of this chapter you will be able to:

- Use some tools to help raise self-awareness
- Start to consider how being self-aware can help us work with patients/ clients/service users
- Think about how your values, thoughts and feelings impact on your support work role
- Apply a model of reflection.

Setting the scene

Working in the health care and/or social care sector is challenging. Professionally and personally, you will experience the high and lows of delivering care and support to those in need if you choose support work as a career. The highs from delivering care and support are generally easier to handle, pro-fessionally and personally. Helping another human being can be a wonderful, life-affirming experience. Providing care and support to others can validate the version of ourselves we hope others will see. We are thanked by clients and their families, they shake our hands, shed tears of gratitude and send us cards and flowers. However, we must also be prepared for the lows: the clients and family members who do not have happy outcomes, or who are unhappy with their care, or who simply do not like us and nothing we do will change that fact.

Outside the world of support work and the professional helping relationship, your own personal life continue its course. You will experience positive and negative life events that will leave their mark: relationships, both good and bad, births, deaths, house moves. Sometimes, the positives events happen in quick succession, and, sometimes, the negative events seem to dominate and can overwhelm us and make us feel weaker versions of ourselves. All of life will impact on your day-to-day work and 'ways of being' as a support worker caring for people.

Being self-aware

> Self-awareness skills involve exploration of thoughts, feelings, behaviours.
>
> (Sharples 2013, p. 206)

Future chapters will touch on 'ethical practice', but in this chapter we want you to stop for a moment and look in the mirror and consider the person you see, reflected back at you.

Today, working people are living very busy lives; trying to balance respon-sibilities and rushing home from work to manage hectic personal lives, we can find it hard to take stock of things. The following activity is designed to help you to stop and think a little about how things are for you now, in this moment. The wheel of life is commonly used in the field of coaching to raise awareness. This is the first activity of the book; please look at the example and then read the instructions and follow the steps in the activity box.

Box 2.1 Activity: Wheel of life activity to raise awareness

Step 1: Find a blank piece of paper and draw a circle in the centre of the page. The whole circle represents your life at this moment in time.

Step 2: You can now divide the circle into equal segments; Figure 2.1 is an example. Label segments so they meaningfully apply to your life. You can add as segments as you wish, but make all the segments equal.

Step 3: Consider each segment separately and, using a 0–10 scale, rate each segment according to the level of satisfaction you feel about it: 0 = completely dissatisfied, 10 = completely satisfied.

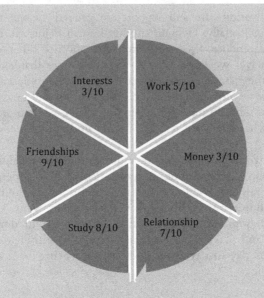

Figure 2.1 The wheel of life
Source: Adapted from Byrne 2005

Step 4: Look at the satisfaction score you have given yourself. Remember that this is a snapshot of how things stand today only. What do you notice looking at the segments and the scores? For example, do you have the same scores in each segment, or are some doing better than others?

Step 5: How do these scores make you feel? You might find that high scores have more positive emotions attached to them, such as happiness and joy, and, therefore, low scores make you feel disappointed and hopeless, even sad. Surprisingly, you might also find that the low scores don't bother you at all.

In the example wheel of life provided in Figure 2.1, there are higher scores in the segments for 'study', 'friendships' and 'relationship', and lower satisfaction scores in areas such as 'interests' and 'money'. It is possible that the example wheel shows a person who is struggling to get the balance of their life right. However, the meaning behind these scores is personal to the person. What issues have your scores raised for you?

In this chapter, we are trying to demonstrate that, as self-aware support workers, we must have a clear understanding of the different parts of our life and also be able to self-assess how the different parts of our lives impact on the helping relationship we offer to patients. Particularly of concern are those parts of our lives that cause us worry and stress, as they could have an impact on the quality of care we provide.

As we can see from the following scenario, life's problems do not necessarily evaporate because we are at work. To be consistent and effective in our care giving and support responsibilities, we need to be able to notice changes in our own emotional state and take responsibility.

Box 2.2 Activity

Care worker Maureen has just checked her bank balance in the car, before a home visit to an older person, Carol. Maureen is very overdrawn, again, and she still has 4 days until payday and lots of outgoings. Maureen is the only person visiting Carol today.

Questions to consider:

What thoughts and feelings might be triggered for Maureen because of her bank balance?

How might the thoughts and feelings impact on her behaviour during the visit with Carol?

The case for understanding how important this self-knowledge is starts with the relationship between you and the client who requires your help. As you will perhaps know by now, clients come from all walks of life; some may familiar to you, and some may be completely outside your own experience and imagination.

It might feel very easy to help clients who are like us. You might feel like you can do your best for them; you get positive feedback that affirms you are well equipped and in control of the situation and can make their life better. It feels good to work with people like ourselves: we can use humour perhaps, and they get our jokes. We can provide advice, and they take it and appreciate we are doing our very best for them. Clients who are unlike ourselves can also be equally rewarding to work with, of course. They offer new and rich learning opportunities, and, as long as they are active in responding to the 'helping relationship', then everything can run smoothly. It has often been considered to be of primary importance that the worker possesses excellent communication skills in all contexts and with every client, but this is challenging, exhausting and unrealistic when working in pressured environments with limited resources. Self-awareness and self-knowledge can help you to notice the relationships you have with patients and seek help and support when needed.

Emotional intelligence

Maureen, Carol's support worker, is now flooded with anxiety about her current overdraft but she is going to see an older person who is socially isolated and needs her to be able to listen and put her at the centre of the visit. Maureen needs, therefore, to be present in mind and body for Carol.

Emotional intelligence is 'the ability to monitor one's own and others' feelings and emotions, to discriminate among them and to use this information to guide one's thinking and actions' (Salovey and Mayer 1990, p. 189). It has become the focus of considerable interest in health and social care (Birks and Watt 2007). Traditionally, it has been thought that the health and social care professional was trained sufficiently to be able to switch off or put aside their uncomfortable emotions/feelings within the caring context and perform using the more rational part of their brain. The public had faith in the belief that the professional would be equipped to offer stable delivery of care, and each patient would be treated the same. There is now an acknowledgement in training that it is important to recognise our emotions, alongside having the skill of being able to notice the emotions of patients. Just checking on ourselves, every day, and asking 'How am I today?' might be worthwhile.

Box 2.3 Advice

What advice would you offer Maureen before she goes into Carol's house to provide care?
  Example advice:

- Take a few deep breaths before you go into the house.
- Remind yourself that you can worry about the money problem after your home visit with Carol, which is in an hour's time.

The Johari window

The Johari window is a self-development tool developed by two psychologists, Joseph Luft and Harrington Ingham, in the early 1960s. The Johari window is still used today in many different professional and personal development contexts, including health and social care. The four quadrants draw attention to the 'known' and 'unknown' parts of ourselves. Using the tool can help you start to raise awareness about the parts of yourself that you and others know about and those parts of you that others might have some awareness of, but you don't. The areas in the quadrant that can raise the most concern in a caring relationship are those we and others might be blind to because we have no awareness of them or they are not an important part of what we value in the day-to-day.

In order to use the Johari window effectively, you are required to have a conversation with those who know you to help build awareness. We suggest you start with yourself by filling in the box that is 'known' to you and then share with your own close social network of family and friends and see what you learn about yourself that you didn't know. However, it is also important that people in your network understand that you want to be able to make positive changes as a consequence of the discussion and that this is to enhance how you help people in your work role and responsibilities. If you look at the example of Morgan, a healthcare support worker, in Figure 2.2, you can see that she is unaware of her behaviour towards patients when she goes without food; this is a resolvable issue.

Discrimination

What sometimes can be 'unknown' to ourselves is how we respond to people who are different to us; this is called 'unconscious bias'. Since we started this book, there have been two major movements that have led to international public protests (peaceful and violent), high-profile court cases and debates within academia, the international media and social media. The Me Too campaign and the Black Lives Matter campaign have forced many people around the world to face uncomfortable truths about their previous responses to witnessing discrimination, whether racial, sexual or other forms. In support work, you will work with 'diversity' in your client groups and you will be expected to act if you witness discriminatory behaviour.

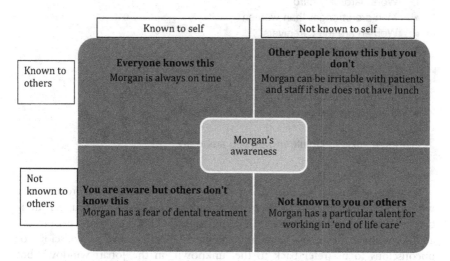

Figure 2.2 Johari window example for healthcare support worker Morgan
Source: Adapted from Luft (1984)

Box 2.4 Prompting questions

What might be hidden from you but others can see because of:

- Your gender?
- Your sexuality?
- Your ethnicity?
- Your social class?
- Your abilities?
- Your spiritual beliefs?

Can you add to this list?

Values and beliefs

The stoic philosopher Epictetus is supposed to have said these words: 'Men are disturbed not by things, but by the views which they take of things'.

Our view of things or our perspective on things can be based on the values or rules we live our life by, not necessarily based on either fact or truth, until, again, we get asked questions about them.

Box 2.5 Values

- Family is everything
- Money makes everything better
- Work hard/play hard
- Men are stronger than women
- Women are the caregivers
- Children need discipline
- Respect your elders
- Change is exciting
- My values are informed by my faith
- If you work hard you can achieve everything

List three values that inform who you are today.

Looking at the list in Box 2.5, you might have nodded in agreement or winced and considered a couple of items very controversial and found it difficult to comprehend anyone else holding those beliefs. However, people do, and sometimes they may be your patients. Our values maybe conscious or unconscious to us (refer back to the 'unknown' in the Johari window), but either way values can reveal themselves in our interactions with others without us knowing. We can, therefore, be judged or we become the judges, or both.

The impact of this in a helping/caring relationship is worth considering. In the world outside the caring role, we often make the decision to remove ourselves from those who are not like us. In caring roles, however, we must move towards people who do not share our values and demonstrate empathy and compassion towards them. It is, therefore, essential that we try to understand what might get in the way of being able to do this.

Reflection in action

Learning how to reflect on ourselves while working in health and social care practice is a core part of the curriculum of most courses in the field. By learning the art of reflection, it is hoped, the practitioner will consciously engage in a structured process that supports them in actively learning from events and experiences. Being a 'reflective practitioner' can help you develop both professionally and personally. However, being reflective involves time and space to consider how we think, behave and feel in situations that can challenge us. Within the health and social care literature, this has been written about extensively, and there are countless models out there. If you ask your professional colleagues which reflective models they use to support their continuing professional development, they would probably refer to one of the following: Gibbs (1988), Johns (2004) or Kolb (1984). Schon (1995) described reflection as the 'swampy lowlands', which shows how challenging it is to even describe.

For the purposes of this textbook, we have chosen Gibbs's (1988) reflective cycle; it is commonly used in practice, but also in learning environments to enable students to structure their reflective assignments. We also chose Gibbs because, as you can see from Figure 2.3, the cycle requests that you are

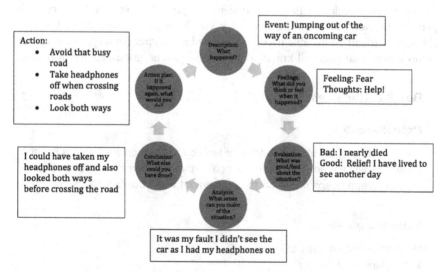

Figure 2.3 An adapted example of Gibb's (1988) reflective cycle in action

prompted to consider your feelings, alongside your thinking. This model therefore tunes into the emotional dimension of the helping experience. For example, if you think about split second decisions you have made in your life, the feeling might have been what prompted you into action with no time for a thought, so feelings are very powerful and do stay with us when we recall something significant.

Box 2.6 Activity

Apply Gibb's reflective cycle to your own significant event. Make sure you work through all the stages to conclude with a meaningful action plan.

Support work practice requires us to be active in reflection for the safety and care of patients and clients. Reflection should not be a comfortable process either; it should force us to ask ourselves some difficult questions about our shortcomings as well as help us identify our strengths and our own areas for development and need; otherwise, at best, our practice remains unchanged or, at worst, we make mistakes that can cause harm to our clients. None of us is perfect, and, as the high-profile cases we hear about in the media illustrate, serious mistakes are made.

A way of helping you see from the patient's perspective using reflection involves you recalling your own experiences/memories of what it felt like when you or your loved ones have been patients or clients. In this book, we call this the 'I' test. The 'I' test activity requires you to think about experiences from the first-person perspective of being a patient and/or carer in order to gain knowledge and understanding.

The NHS, founded in 1948, was designed to provide healthcare 'from cradle to grave'. Therefore, it would be unusual if you have escaped any contact with it, although it might be possible if you were raised in another country. However, the authors argue that you will know, as a potential patient, good practice from bad.

Box 2.7 The 'I' test

Reflective activity

Try to think of a significant event that led you to have contact with a health and/or social care service or professional, either for yourself or a loved one – for example, a hospital visit or an appointment with your GP.

Reflective questions

What your first impression?
What stands out to you?
What was positive about the experience?

- What did you think?
- What did you feel?
- What did you do?

What was negative about the experience?

- What did you think?
- What did you feel?
- What did you do?

Stonehouse (2014, p. 397) argues that support workers are 'ideally placed', because of their focus on the relationship, to 'support and facilitate good quality communication in the workplace'; however, the support worker also needs to be able to identify the barriers to communication that clients and their families experience and work hard to try to remove them.

Self-awareness and recognising the negative toll of caring

'Burn-out' and 'compassion fatigue' are concepts that are researched and talked about in the caring professions. Burn-out has been defined by Yang and Hayes (2020, p. 1) as 'a psychological syndrome characterised by emotional exhaustion, depersonalisation, and a reduced sense of personal accomplishment'. Burn-out is the opposite of feeling you have energy, motivation and a desire to do the best for the people you work with; it can be linked to compassion fatigue, which can happen in the moment with patients and obviously means that you will lose the ability to connect with them (Yang and Hayes 2020). Self-awareness is key for the support worker to be able to recognise the signs and be able to take steps to provide good care. Neither burn-out nor compassion fatigue are necessarily a reflection of you being a bad practitioner (although this might be the case); instead, it might be that the demands made on you in your workplace exceed your ability to cope. To put this in perspective, some health and social care professionals have a very short career expectancy post qualification owing to the demands of their role; this can be because they carry large caseloads and are exposed to trauma and even risk of violence. Self -awareness is necessary for some of us to be able to see the signs. Burn-out is a concern in the caring professions and in organisations where staff face high demands but also have limited resources as they strive to do their job to the best of their ability. Be warned, however: burn-out is not easily recognisable for the individual. If you refer back to the Johari window, it might be in the quadrant that is hidden to you and possibly to your team and organisation. However, the organisation you work for has a duty of care to ensure your health and safety, and excellent supervision and peer support can really help here. It is entirely normal to have good days and bad days at work; however, some of these signs, experienced in a sustained way, can compromise the way care is experienced by the patient, and they are at the centre of all we do.

Box 2.8 Checklist of signs of burn out

- Tiredness
- Feeling exhausted
- Poor motivation
- Making less effort
- Taking no interest in patients or clients
- Depression
- Disconnect from patients and colleagues.

Supervision and mentoring

> Supervision is any activity where more experienced health professionals provide less experienced health professionals with opportunities that enable these health professionals to achieve learning, to receive support, and to improve the quality and safety of their practice.
>
> (Fitzpatrick et al. 2012, p. 462)

In your current workplace, how much time do you get to reflect on your own practice in a focused conversation? You may be fortunate enough to have an excellent, clearly scheduled supervision timetable, or you may have a more informal arrangement, or you might not have any at all. Supervision and mentoring provide a way for you to learn your role and extend your skills. Good supervision can offer you professional development opportunities too. A good supervisor will understand that your own well-being is important, notice signs of stress and be supportive of you engaging in activities to enhance self-awareness, and this will directly impact on the quality of care provided. However, there can be barriers to getting good supervision. Do you recognise any of these in the organisation you work in?

Table 2.1 Checklist of signs and symptoms of compassion fatigue

Physical	Emotional	Work-related
Headaches	Moody	Avoiding working with patients
Heart problems	Easily irritated	Not caring as much about patients or their families
Can't sleep or sleep too much	Can't concentrate	Taking lots of sick days
	Can't remember things easily	Not liking the job anymore

Source: Adapted from Lombardo and Eyre 2011, p. 3

Peer support

In health and social care, we often look to the person above us in the hierarchy for guidance and support – a manager or qualified professional. However, seeking support from our peers is another avenue available to us. People in roles similar to ours can be useful for our own professional development and self-awareness. However, the skill is to choose the right person(s) who will support you positively to move forward in your role so that you can improve your work with clients. These people might offer you more informal guidance, perhaps in those rare moments when you have time for a cup of tea and a catch-up.

Box 2.9 Qualities to look for in a peer support supervisor

- They model a commitment to the 6 Cs.
- Clients and family feedback are positive.
- Respected by colleagues in their team.
- They invest in their own continuing professional development.
- They model self-awareness and self-care.

Resilience

> To be able to overcome stressors or withstand negative life events and, not only recover from such experiences, but also find personal meaning in them (Klohen, 1996; Youssef and Luthans, 2007).
>
> (Grant and Kinman 2012, p. 605)

Resilience has become a popular word in the field. You might have heard managers talking about building team resilience, or there may even be training to attend in your organisation. Resilience is the capacity to cope with difficult/ stressful events and bounce back from them, and Grant and Kinman (2012) suggest that you have the capacity to move on and feel that the tough time added something to your life experience. It is a concept that is applied to organisations as well as the individuals and teams working within them. There is no doubt that, in this resource-thin time in health and social care, a support worker will have to 'dig deep'.

Box 2.10 Reflective exercise

Think of a tough time in your life.
  Questions:

- How did you cope with this?
- Are you happy with how you coped?
- Do you reflect on the event as something that, although unfortunate or unhappy, provided you with a sense of growth?

Self–care

'Physician, heal thyself.' You have probably heard this phrase. It wisely suggests doctors take care of themselves before they advise patients how to. Carl Jung, founder of analytic psychology, also warned of the 'wounded healer', and this concept has been adopted subsequently in health and social care. The idea that those attracted to the helping relationship may also have 'wounds' they live with has been researched in healthcare. You are at risk of the same, as the nature of support work can take its toll on your emotional, physical and social well-being. You work with vulnerable people whom you may support to wash, eat, drink, access leisure, see family and pay their bills. How about you? Are you able to achieve a balance in your own life? The wheel of life might have shown you a few things to attend to and you may have let things slip. We can often blame ourselves in these situations, but the reasons are more complex, especially in the demanding sectors of health and social care.

Another helpful and much referred to tool is Maslow's hierarchy of needs (1968), often used by those working in health and social care to consider the needs of patients. However, applying Maslow's hierarchy to our own lives might also reveal gaps. Maslow's hierarchy is commonly depicted as a pyramid, with a broad base that has human beings' physiological requirements for survival – such as food, sleep, warmth, shelter – at the bottom. The next layer contains 'safety' needs: as human beings, in order to survive and thrive, Maslow suggests we need to be physically and emotionally safe. As the pyramid narrows, the next layer contains belonging and love, which we might find in partnerships, family and friends. The last two elements – esteem needs and self-actualisation – are really the icing on the cake for human beings. Esteem is linked to being valued by those around us, and, finally, if we can 'self-actualise' we can be who we want to be in our lives.

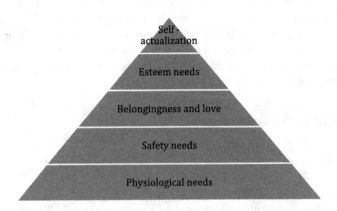

Figure 2.4 Adapted Maslow's hierarchy of needs
Source: Maslow 1968

Box 2.11 Activity: Try applying Maslow's hierarchy to John

John works as a support worker for children with complex needs in the community. He does regular night shifts. He has recently separated from his wife and is currently homeless, although he described it as 'sofa surfing' to his manager. He is providing financial support for all three of his children who now live with his estranged wife and he has little money left at the end of the month. He is creeping into debt.

What happens if John comes to work to find two of his colleagues have gone off sick and his manager is suggesting that John has room to increase his own caseload to cover the absences? This means squeezing in more home visits into what is already a tough working week.

Where would you locate John on Maslow's hierarchy of needs?

How might John's circumstances be impacting on his mental and physical well-being?

How might John's circumstances impact on the care he provides for the children he works with:

- Physically?
- Emotionally?
- Socially?

Conclusion

Being responsive to clients' needs is a central part of the support worker role and helps you build a rapport and maintain the relationship. The important point we are making by offering tools such as reflective models, the wheel of life, the Johari window and Maslow's hierarchy is that, as a support worker, your past and present circumstances, alongside the training and experience in the field, will influence how you carry out your role and how you will make use of the responsibility and power it gives you to work with vulnerable people.

In this chapter, we hope to have convinced you that building your self-awareness is part of the toolkit you need to be a reflective practitioner. By engaging in the exercises, you will have noticed that your values, thoughts, feelings and past and present experiences do not get washed away as you take on the responsibilities of a support worker: they inform who you can be, as a support worker, for better or for worse.

References

Birks, Y.F. and Watt, I.S. (2007). Emotional intelligence and patient-centred care. *Journal of the Royal Society of Medicine*, 100, 368–374.

Byrne, U. (2005). Work–life balance: Why are we talking about it at all? *Business Information Review*, 22(1), 53–59.

Fitzpatrick, S., Smith, M., and Wilding, C. (2012). Quality allied health clinical supervision policy in Australia: A literature review. *Australian Health Review*, 36, 461–465.

Gibbs, G. (1988). *Learning by doing: A guide to teaching and learning methods*. Oxford: Further Education Unit, Oxford Polytechnic.

Grant, L. and Kinman, G. (2012). Enhancing wellbeing in social work students: Building resilience in the next generation. *Social Work Education*, 31(5), 605–621.

Henson S.J. (2020). Burnout or compassion fatigue: A comparison of concepts. *MEDSURG Nursing (MEDSURG NURS)*, 29(2), 77–95.

Johns, C. (2004). *Becoming a reflective practitioner* (2nd ed.). Oxford: Blackwell Publishing.

Klohen, E. (1996). Conceptual analysis and measurement of the construct of ego resiliency. *Journal of Personality and Social Psychology*, 70(5), 1067–1079.

Kolb, D.A. (1984). *Experiential learning: Experience as the source of learning and development* (Vol. 1). Englewood Cliffs, NJ: Prentice-Hall.

Lombardo, B. and Eyre, C. (2011). Compassion fatigue: A nurse's primer. *Online Journal of Nursing*, 16(1), 3. doi:10.3912/OJIN.Vol16No01Man03

Luft, J. (1984). *Group process: An introduction to group dynamics* (3rd ed.). New York: McGraw Hill.

Maslow, A. (1968). *Towards a psychology of being* (2nd ed.). Toronto: Van Nostrand.

Salovey, P. and Mayer, J.D. (1990). Emotional intelligence. *Imagination, Cognition and Personality*, 9(3), 185–211.

Schon, D. (1995). *The reflective practitioner: How professionals think in action*. Aldershot, UK: Arena.

Sharples, N. (2013). Relationship, helping and communication skills. In: Brooker, C. and Waugh, A. (eds), *Foundations of nursing practice*. Edinburgh: Mosby Elsevier, 221–250.

Stonehouse, D. (2014). Communication and the support worker. *British Journal of Healthcare Assistants*, 08(08), 394–397.

Yang, Y. and Hayes, J.A. (2020). Causes and consequences of burnout among mental health professionals: A practice-oriented review of recent empirical literature. *Psychotherapy*. Advance online publication. http://dx.doi.org/10.1037/pst0000317

Youssef, Y. and Luthans, F. (2007). Positive organizational behaviour in the workplace: The impact of hope, optimism and resilience. *Journal of Management*, 33, 774–800.

3 Know your support worker role

Paul Mackreth

Introduction

The previous chapter of this handbook will have helped you to understand yourself better through understanding what it means to be 'self-aware'. You will have understood that being self-aware can enable you to be more person-centred as a support worker. Support work in health and social care is about human interaction, and we use our awareness of self as a tool to care for others.

This chapter builds upon your knowledge of self by asking you to learn and understand your own support worker role. You may argue that you understand your role as it is what you do on a day-to-day basis – who else should understand your role better than you? We do not dispute this. The aim of this chapter is to facilitate you being able to explain what health and social care support work is. In this chapter, and others, we use the term 'context' as it means that it looks at the bigger picture, of which, we argue, you are an important part.

To do this, we will detail the scope of the role and the different names and titles that are used under the umbrella of 'support work'. You will be surprised at the breadth of the role. It may even give you ideas for your own career pathway (see Chapter 9). We will look at what studies have found in terms of the number of support workers in the United Kingdom, where they work and how much they get paid! We will also detail some issues in terms of the value of the role. We think you will agree that there have been times when you have been valued and times when you have not been valued. We conclude with our belief that, by understanding the 'context' of your role, you will be able to articulate how valuable your role is in the delivery of health and social care. We know that you know this already, but can you explain it to others?

Box 3.1 Quiz

How many support workers are there in the UK?
How many titles do they use?
What is the average rate of pay for a support worker in the NHS?
... And in social care?

Answers follow in this chapter.

Learning outcomes

At the end of this chapter you will be able to:

- Describe the generic title of 'support worker' and why it is used
- Detail the scope of your practice and what you need to learn to make changes to your practice
- Compare your role to other support worker roles
- Articulate the value that you bring to person-centred care
- Start to consider making connections with other support workers who work with the same clients that you do.

Setting the scene

The background to the support worker role is varied and complex. We should start this discussion with the most important person, the patient/client. We now know that client needs are changing. Changes in our communities mean that there are now more people who are living longer, and that these people are likely to have more than one health condition (NHS England 2019). The result is that there are more people who need care and support, and these people have more complex issues. This is just one aspect of a rapidly increasing demand for services across health, social and charitable care. There are many other issues, such as migration, loss of family support, increasing demands upon carers and lifestyle changes, that other textbooks devote their pages to (the NHS England 2019 Long Term Plan details these challenges very well) and are beyond the scope of this chapter. What we need to realise is that the demand for our services is rapidly increasing, and there are lots of agencies who are working together to create strategies to meet these demands (e.g. NHS England 2019).

The traditional picture of a doctor, nurse, occupational therapist, physiotherapist or social worker providing care is changing; it has had to. Qualified staff, often called 'professionals', are not able to provide all of the care or support that is needed. They either have other duties/demands placed upon them or they are in short supply. Increasingly, the demand for care has outstripped the supply of services and this has forced changes in practice (Royal College of

Nursing Policy Unit 2009; NHS England 2014; NHS England 2019; Maybin, Charles and Honeyman 2016).

'Skill mix' is a term that has been used for a long time to describe how it is more cost-effective and a better use of skills for people to provide care based upon their skills. Some experts (Aiken et al. 2017) argue that this may be a 'dilution' of roles, and that it does not always lead to quality health and social care. However, the reality is that this is now common across all areas of public life. We see in our own personal lives police community support officers who have effectively supported the police in community policing; teaching assistants are now part of every school classroom; and we see physician assistants in GP surgeries.

Box 3.2 Activity: The role of a health visitor

Think about the role of a health visitor. The health visitor provides community health advice and monitoring for babies and their families. A key part of their role is to monitor the weight of a baby to see if they are thriving: they simply weigh the baby and record the weight. Is a highly qualified health visitor needed to do this, or could other support workers undertake this role?

- Who do you think can weigh a baby?
- What skills and knowledge would this worker require?
- What reporting structure would need to be in place?

Health visitors argue that they can provide the whole package of care, but this may limit their time in other, more complex family cases such as where issues of safety have been raised. Who else may be able to weigh the baby? Who else is qualified to monitor baby well-being?

Your role may be one of the newer 'skill-mixed' support worker roles, or it may be a role that patients and clients are much more used to, such as auxiliary nurse, healthcare assistant or social care assistant. What is clear is that support worker roles are increasingly popular. This is not about reducing the cost of health and social care, but the need to find adequate numbers of staff. The demand for care means that there are not enough 'professional staff', and their time is increasingly taken up with the assessment of care. So, does an organisation such as the NHS or a local authority wait 3–4 years for a new nurse, midwife, social worker, occupational therapist or dietitian to fill a vacant post, or do they look at 'skill mix' to employ a support worker, where possible, and train them to a minimum standard in 12 weeks?

Box 3.3 Activity: Example of workforce numbers: district nurses

We use the example of district nurse as it is a well-established role that is common across the UK. It is a role that is central in delivering care at home through a team of community nurses. They are part of the wider nursing workforce that has a shortfall of more than 41,000 nurses across the NHS (QNI 2019).

The numbers of district nurses have been dropping for several years, despite the NHS calling for a more community care-led NHS (Department of Health 2005; NHS England 2019). In 2003, there were 12,620 district nurses; in 2013, this was down to 6,656 (National Nurses Research Unit 2013). In 2019, the Queens Nursing Institute highlighted that numbers have continued to drop and found that (in England) they were down to approximately 4,000. That's for a population of more than 55 million.

So, who is now providing the care?

There are lots of questions and debates about this. Some are ethical and moral (what is right and wrong) questions. These questions have been brought into sharp focus by high-profile cases of abuse where support workers have perpetrated crimes relating to abuse (e.g. Winterbourne View). What follows is a review of just some of these issues that we feel you should understand to do your job better.

Your title

As we have indicated in the introduction to this book, we use the umbrella term 'support work' for many roles across health and social care; this includes the many charities and other organisations that offer services, not just the NHS and local authorities. Just like the traditional picture of who is providing care, the traditional picture of where care takes place is changing. Since the National Health Service and Community Care Act (1990), there has been a government policy to move care away from hospital settings into the community. We must, therefore, acknowledge the breadth of community, health and social care services. This means that support work is not just the role of the worker who supports nurses on a hospital ward, but a whole host of other areas that mean a lot to clients.

Box 3.4 Support worker example: Alex, Healthy Homes

When Alex was younger, he realised that he liked to help people: he used to help a neighbour on his street with things such as getting the mail or shopping. Alex decided that he would like to have a career where he can help others. He now works with Healthy Homes. He has the title 'support worker' and acts as an advocate for his clients, who suffer from mental health issues. He attends case conferences with his clients, assists them to understand what is being discussed and speaks for his clients when needed. Although his employer used to be a housing association, it is clear that people who need assistance with housing often have other health problems. This is Alex's role.

If you are asking ,'So, with so many roles and settings to work in, how can we all be termed under one umbrella of support work?', then you are asking the right question. Kessler et al. (2010) wrote a comprehensive history and tried to define the different, evolving support roles. They only wrote about the hospital setting but highlighted that there are issues with different workplaces having different practices, role definitions and job descriptions. However, they indicated that, if the workforce was brought together under a unified title of 'support workers', there might be more than 1 million support workers across the United Kingdom. This would make them the largest workforce in health-care. Moran, Enderby and Nancarrow (2010) supported this assertion, high-lighting that, despite some differences, they should be viewed as the largest workforce in healthcare.

Since these papers were published, the government undertook and published the Cavendish Review (2013). This was a significant report by Camilla Cavendish, who was an editor at *The Times* newspaper and a health advisor to the prime minister. She led 'an independent review into healthcare assistants and support workers in the NHS and social care settings'. She also found that there are vast numbers of staff who are in support work roles and suggested that the figure might be around 1.3 million, but that it is not absolutely possible to quantify as roles can be very different. In the report, she presented some key facts (2013, p. 13) that are shown in Table 3.1.

Box 3.5 Activity: Key facts

Have a look at Table 3.1. Do you recognise your role in this chart? Do consider that some of these facts are now quite old, but do they look similar?

Box 3.6 Activity: Support worker job titles

Can you list as many different support worker job titles as possible? How many can you get? (Tip: if you include technician roles, then you will get a longer list.)

Kessler et al. (2010) also discussed that the job titles given to support workers are often rooted in the differing professional groups that they support. Herber and Johnston (2013) identified 30 titles used in health, and Moran et al. (2010) produced an exhaustive table of 75 titles used for support roles in healthcare.

Table 3.1 Key statistics for healthcare assistants and support workers

	Health	Social care
Size of workforce		
	160,500 (2012 narrowest definition) 332,000 (Francis 2013; comprising 270,000 providing support for doctors and nurses and 62,000 among the scientific and technical staff)	1,225 million (2011)
Demographic information		
Gender	84% female	84% female
Ethnicity (Black and minority ethnic groups)	15%	29%
Average age	45	35 (new starters, with no evidence of an ageing workforce)
Where do they work?		
	>50% in the acute sector (acute, elderly, general)	Almost 50% in domiciliary care (providing care in a person's home)
How long do they remain in the post?		
Average number of years in the post	4.1 (average across England)	59% spend between 2 and 6 years in the post, with 29% having been in the post for no more than 6 years
Turnover and pay		
Turnover	14%	£19.8%
Pay	56% paid between £14,249 and £17,425 pa (Agenda for Change Band 2)	£13,974 pa (average)

Source: Adapted from Cavendish 2013, n.p.

Changing roles and your duty of care

Box 3.7 Activity: How has your role changed?

How much has your role changed since you started it? What do you do now that you did not do at the start of your role or in the last 12 months?

We are sure that you will agree that your role has changed a lot since it commenced. You will have taken on more duties, as well as more responsibility. The number of people you are responsible for might have grown, as well as there being change in the range of work you do with them. You will also be doing a variety of different work with your clients. The Cavendish Report (2013) was clear that support workers are taking on more tasks, and that some of these are highly advanced.

Box 3.8 Activity: Complex/advanced care

The authors do not consider 'basic care' to mean 'easy care', as care giving requires complex human interaction However, there are some aspects of care that are more complex than others. What do you do in your role that could be described as 'complex' or 'advanced'? For example, we have met support workers who look after children who are on home ventilation via a tracheostomy and, in some situations, they need to change the tracheostomy tube. While they are doing this, the child is unable to breathe until the tube is placed back in! Other support workers help people to recover after they have tried to take their own lives. But are these skills any more advanced than washing someone who is unwell? They all need the skills of compassion, trust and communication. Write down what you think is complex and challenging about your work.

Moran, Nancarrow, Enderby and Bradburn (2012) write that this is 'extending' your practice. They believe that this has implications for both you and the people that you work with. They use the term 'boundaries for practice'. Other authors also write about boundaries in practice in fields such as palliative care (Ingleton, Chatwin, Seymour and Payne 2011), maternity care (Griffin, Dunkley-Bent, Skewes and Linay 2010) and primary care and in the intermediate care setting (Galloway and Smith 2005).

In many cases, you accept care delegated to you, working 'under' professional staff (Lloyd-Jones 2008). However, expanding your role to undertake tasks previously the remit of 'qualified' professionals results in you being more independent and having to make independent decisions (Hand 2010; Skills for Health 2011). If this is the case, then you must consider that you are accountable and must work to a code of practice (Hussain and Marshall 2011).

Box 3.9 Activity: Code of practice

Do you know about the support worker code of practice? Have you read it? If you live in Northern Ireland (Northern Ireland Social Care Council n.d.), Wales (GIG Cymru/NHS Wales n.d.) or Scotland (NHS Scotland 2009), you have your own country-specific code. You must read your code. What does the section on 'accountability' make you think with regards to the work that you take on?

High-profile safeguarding issues in support work practice has led to minimum core principles of practice published in these codes of practice. Despite the differences in support worker roles, research does show that there are core aspects of practice (Moran et al. 2010; Baldwin et al. 2003), allowing for the development of these generic standards for care.

A key recommendation of the 2013 Cavendish Report is that all support workers have a minimum amount of training. We now see this in the 'care certificate' (Skills for Health n.d.) that you would have completed if you are working in a support role.

Your employer's duty

Although you should always consider that you are accountable for accepting duties and then delivering the care and support, your employer also has a duty. For the reasons listed earlier in this chapter, health and social care organisations have reviewed their workforce in favour of support workers roles and have further developed new, more autonomous 'assistant' or 'associate' roles (Skills for Health 2011; Nursing and Midwifery Council 2018). They argue this will lead to more effective and responsive client-focused care.

Some writers (Moran et al. 2012) are critical and suggest that the roles are not fully understood, and so support worker skills are not deployed effectively. Other authors (Kessler et al. 2010) highlight the potential for conflict between support workers and health professionals given the rapid expansion in support roles that could be viewed as role 'substitution', rather than role 'support' of a registered practitioner. Moran et al. (2012) confirmed this tension and encourage health managers to overcome tensions given the imperative for workforce change. Despite these challenges, the expansion of support worker roles and the introduction of new 'associate' roles remain a key part of health service modernisation (NHS Employers 2010; NHS England 2019).

To address some of these issues, organisations should now be providing more in-house training for support workers (Herber and Johnston 2013). Much of this is rooted in competency frameworks that demand an expansion of the support workers' skills to expand their scope of practice (Rolf et al. 1999; Hussain and Marshall 2011). These build on the care certificate and ensure that any expansion of a role is 'assured' to keep care safe.

It is now commonplace for support workers only to be 'allowed' to undertake procedures once they have been 'signed off' as being competent. This competency process is also linked to certain client groups (on pathways of care) and certain situations (against set protocols) – see Chapter 8 for more detail. It is significant, as practice has not always been like this, but employers use these tools to ensure that they provide safe care in practice for which they are accountable.

You should question any organisation that asks you to do something that you have never had training in, and, once it is understood that you are not trained to do a task, it should not be undertaken.

Moral duty

You will see from Chapter 2 that we use the word 'ethics' and understand that ethics are about different interpretations of what is right and wrong. Ethics, however, are a very complex issue, as what is right for one person is often wrong for another. Ethics are, therefore, a complex area of philosophy that is defined by its study of 'morality'. In terms of health and social care, ethics are often described as 'medical ethics'. There are some high-profile cases where medical ethics have been so complicated that the high courts have been needed to decide for us.

Box 3.10 Activity: Right to die

Search the internet (news sections) for 'right to die'. You will see that there are some very complex cases with very different views. You will have your own view. This view will often be part of how you practise your role.

We believe (and this is well covered in lots of textbooks, as well as in your code of conduct) that it is important to think about this on a day-to-day basis. It is good practice to consider what is right or wrong to ensure that we do not do harm. Sadly, the history of health and social care practice is full of occasions where people have done harm when they thought that they were doing good.

Mental health care, in particular, is well illustrated as doing harm to patients in the goal of 'making them better'. The asylums were built and designed to give people rest and to be places of sanctuary, but, if you think of the word 'asylum' now in relation to mental health, you will have an image of them being places of harm, with visions of gothic horror movies, inhumane treatments and torture. When you talk to patients who were admitted to the old asylums, some people did not like them, but many also did as they were places to get away from stress.

Some medical testing was thought of as 'routine' in the 1990s, until people started questioning it. In England, we saw parents of children who had died discovering that their dead child's organs had been retained for medical testing *without* consent. Only after investigation was the true scale of this discovered (see Royal Liverpool Children's Inquiry 2001). We have learned many lessons from these cases, but we also continue to discover or look back on what has happened in health and social care and be shocked.

More recent history has exposed numerous cases, often in social care work, of poor care: see Box 3.11.

Box 3.11 Activity: Cases of abuse

Go to the BBC News web pages and search 'care assistant' in the news section. How many cases of abuse can you read about? What motivated the care assistants to become abusers?

George Orwell wrote a famous essay in 1948 called 'In Front of Your Nose'. In it, he argues that we need to constantly remind ourselves what is right and wrong, and that this takes 'constant struggle'. In his case, it was finding himself thinking negatively about immigration to the UK when, in fact, in the 1940s, just like now, this ignores the complexity of immigration.

If you are to know your own practice, this needs time and space for you to think and write about it (if you find writing helpful). Orwell advocated the keeping of a daily diary so that you can reflect upon your thoughts. This is the same activity that theorists consider good practice in healthcare to ensure that we continually learn from our experience (see Chapter 2, section on reflection).

Box 3.12 Activity: Past practice

As we often look back at the past and think 'I can't believe that we used to do that', can you identify anything about your current practice where you may end up looking back and thinking the same? For example, in the practice of home care, we now know that 15-minute visits to provide care are both ineffective and unpleasant for clients.

Client group

As we will cite many times in this book, our most important goal is to work effectively with clients to assure person–centred care. One thing that we have found in our practice is that, sometimes, 'professional staff' miss the obvious with clients, and your role as a support worker is to speak up or advocate on behalf of your clients. The literature asserts that support workers demonstrate high levels of insight in care delivery and invest time and emotion in their work (Herber and Johnston 2013; Ingleton et al. 2011). Ingleton et al. (2011) suggests this is owing to your proximity to the public, as opposed to the professional distance of the healthcare professions.

Box 3.13 Example: Luke

When Luke worked on a hospital ward, he was in charge of a bay of six patients. Two health care assistants he worked with kept saying that a patient was 'not right', but the patient's observations were stable, and he couldn't objectively see what they were alluding to. However, these health care assistants intuitively knew something was amiss. As the events of that day unfolded, they were proved right, and we were able to gain an early medical review. What Luke learned from that day was always to listen to healthcare assistants/support workers.

Although we do write that there are more people with complex conditions who need all of our support, there is a danger that we stereotype them into 'others' who cannot speak, do not have a voice and have no control. There is a lot written about this in the ethical literature and also a lot of health and social care policy to prevent this 'subjugation' of patients – for example, 'No decision about me without me' (Department of Health 2012).

Box 3.14 Activity: What's in a name?

What's in a name? List as many names as you can that are used for your client group. For example, are they clients or patients? Why do we use all these names to 'other' them? Aren't they just people that we work with and alongside?

However, we are sure that you will agree that all clients, patients or however you refer to the group of people that you work with have strengths. It is this that some parts of health and social care policy are suggesting we can work with (the Care Act, 2014). The term 'assets' is being used as a term to describe how we can find these strengths and see if these can be used to overcome challenges. So, very quickly, we will see roles changing to support a person using their strengths to overcome weaknesses.

Box 3.15 Example: John

John has a spinal injury. He has some limited movement in his hands. Although he needs someone with him most of the time to assist with his activities of daily living, his asset is his ability to communicate well and relate to/debate with others. This has given him the ability to use assistive technology to write books, manage his own team of staff and run a business from home. The support worker role is to facilitate this and certainly not to do everything for him.

Increasingly, we are learning to learn from our clients. We value their life stories and need to learn what their needs are from their voice, not from what is presumed by assessment processes. There are some excellent examples of where service users, carers and other people have got together to form groups to advise health and social care. This may be through general practice (GP) forums, through becoming non-executive board members of NHS trusts or through being invited to 'assess' the performance of nursing students. As the main outcome of what we do, we must listen to the service user's voice.

Conclusion

We have established that your role and practice as a support worker is expanding. There are new, innovative roles such as support for victims of domestic violence (Shakesby and Wallace 2012), nutritional health (Le Cornu et al. 2010) and tissue viability (Lloyd-Jones 2008), together with more traditional caring roles such as personal care (Manthorpe et al. 2010) and nursing home care (Baldwin et al. 2003).

Kitson (2001) cites times when health professions have congruence with health policy. It has been argued that support workers are now congruent with policy given the drive for cost efficiency (Royal College of Nursing Policy Unit 2009) and more recently to address some of the workforce challenges (NHS England 2019).

Traditionally, support workers are 'one step up from lay carers' and can bridge the gap between health professionals and clients and carers (Ingleton et al. 2011). However, there are boundaries and challenges to your role and these have been articulated by the Francis Report (2013). Subsequent to its publication, the Council of Deans of Health (2013) and Cavendish (2013) confirmed that there can be issues with the clarity of the role played by support workers that can lead to frustration. Given the size of the workforce, it could be inferred that this will have a significant effect on the quality of care delivered.

All reports cite poor access to education for support workers: this requires standardisation, and this is now starting to happen. However, you will need time and space to start to understand your role better, and we hope that this chapter will start you on your way in wanting to learn more about the wider context of your role.

References

Aiken, L.H., Sloane, D., Griffiths, P., Rafferty, A. M., Bruyneel, L., McHugh, M., Maier, C. B., Moreno-Casbas, T., Ball, J. E., Ausserhofer, D., and Sermeus, W. (2017). Nursing skill mix in European hospitals: Cross-sectional study of the association with mortality, patient ratings, and quality of care. *BMJ Quality & Safety*, 26, 559–568.

Baldwin, J., Roberts, J.D., Fitzpatrick, J.I., While, A., and Cowan, D.T. (2003). The role of the support worker in nursing homes: A consideration of key issues. *Journal of Nursing Management*, 11, 410–420.

Care Act (c 23). (2014). London: HMSO.

Cavendish, C. (2013). The Cavendish Review: An Independent Review into Healthcare Assistants and Support Workers in the NHS and Social Care Settings [Internet]. www.gov.uk/government/uploads/system/uploads/attachment_data/file/212732/Cavendish_Review_ACCESSIBLE_-_FINAL_VERSION_16-7-13.pdf, accessed on 20 August 2013.

Council of Deans of Health. (2013). Healthcare Support Workers in England [Working Paper]. www.councilofdeans.org.uk/wp-content/uploads/2013/07/CoDH-HCSW-5-proposals-for-investing-in-educdev-for-high-quality-care1.pdf

Department of Health. (2005). Creating a Patient-Led NHS: Delivering the NHS Improvement Plan. London: HMSO.

Department of Health. (2012). Liberating the NHS: No Decision about Me, without Me. HMSO, London.

Francis, R. (2013). *Report of the Mid Staffordshire NHS Foundation Trust Public Inquiry.* London: HMSO.

Galloway, J. and Smith, B. (2005). Meeting the education and training needs of rehabilitation support workers. *International Journal of Therapy and Rehabilitation*, 12(5), 195–199.

Griffin, R., Dunkley-Bent, J., Skewes, J., and Linay, D (2010). Development of maternity support workers role in the UK. *British Journal of Midwifery*, 18(4), 243–246.

Hand, T. (2010). Assistant Practitioner Scoping Project. London: Royal College of Nursing.

Herber, O.R. and Johnston, B. M. (2013). The role of healthcare support workers in providing palliative and end-of-life care in the community: A systematic literature review. *Health and Social Care in the Community*, 21(3), 225–235.

Hussain, C. J. and Marshall, J. E. (2011). The effect of the developing role of the maternity support worker on the professional accountability of the midwife. *Midwifery*, 27, 336–341.

Ingleton, C., Chatwin, J., Seymour, J., and Payne, S. (2011). The role of health care assistants in supporting district nurses and family carers to deliver palliative care at home: Findings from an evaluation project. *Journal of Clinical Nursing*, 20, 2043–2052.

Kessler, I., Heron, P., Dopson, S., Magee, H., Swain , D., and Askham, J. (2010). The Nature and Consequences of Support Workers in a Hospital Setting [Internet]. www. sdo.nihr.ac.uk/files/project/155-final-report.pdf, accessed on 2 December 2011.

Kitson, A. L. (2001). Does nurse education have a future? *Nurse Education Today*, 21, 86–96.

Le Cornu, K.A., Halliday, D.A., Swift, L., Ferris, A., and Gatiss, G.A. (2010). The current and future role of the dietetic support worker. *Journal of Human Nutrition and Dietetics*, 23, 230–237.

Lloyd-Jones, M. (2008). Wound assessment: The role of the healthcare support worker. *British Journal of Healthcare Assistants*, 2(3), 124–126.

Maybin, J., Charles, A., and Honeyman, M. (2016). Understanding Quality in District Nursing Services: Learning from Patients, Carers and Staff. London: The Kings Fund.

Manthorpe, J., Martineau, S., Moriarty, J., Hussein, S., and Stevens, M. (2010). Support workers in social care in England: A scoping study. *Health and Social Care in the Community*, 18(3), 316–324.

Moran, A., Enderby, P., and Nancarrow, S. (2010). Defining and identifying common elements of and contextual influences on the roles of support workers in health and social care: A thematic analysis of the literature. *Journal of Evaluation in Clinical Practice*, 17, 1191–1199.

Moran, A., Nancarrow, S., Enderby, P., and Bradburn, M. (2012). Are we using support workers effectively? The relationship between patient and team characteristics and support worker utilisation in older people's community-based rehabilitation services in England. *Health and Social Care in the Community*, 20(5), 537–549.

National Health Service and Community Care Act (c 19). (1990). London: HMSO.

National Nurses Research Unit. (2013). District Nursing – Who Will Care in the Future? [Internet] www.kcl.ac.uk/nursing/research/nnru/policy/Currentissue/Pol icy–Issue-40.pdf, accessed on 19 November 2013.

Nursing and Midwifery Council. (2018). The Code. www.nmc.org.uk/globalassets/site documents/nmc-publications/nmc-code.pdf

NHS Employers. (2010). The Support Workforce: Developing Your Patient-Facing Staff for the Future [Internet]. www.nhsemployers.org/Aboutus/Publications/Docum ents/The%20support%20workforce.pdf, accessed on 20 August 2013.

NHS England. (2014). Five Year Forward View. www.england.nhs.uk/wp-content/ uploads/2014/10/5yfv-web.pdf

NHS England. (2019). The NHS Long Term Plan. www.longtermplan.nhs.uk/ wp-content/uploads/2019/08/nhs-long-term-plan-version-1.2.pdf

NHS Scotland. (2009). Code of Conduct for Healthcare Support Workers. Edinburgh: Scottish Government.

GIG Cymru/NHS Wales. (n.d.). Code of Conduct for Healthcare Support Workers in Wales. www.wales.nhs.uk/nhswalescodeofconductandcodeofpractice

Northern Ireland Social Care Council. (n.d.). Standards of Conduct and Practice for Social Care Workers. https://niscc.info/storage/resources/standards-of-conduct-and-practice-for-social-care-workers-2019-1.pdf

Orwell, G. (1948). In front of your nose. www.orwellfoundation.com/the-orwell-foundation/orwell/essays-and-other-works/in-front-of-your-nose/

QNI. (2019). Outstanding Models of District Nursing. www.qni.org.uk/wp-content/up loads/2019/05/Oustanding-Models-of-District-Nursing-Report-web.pdf

Rolf, G., Jackson, N., Gardner, L., Jasper, M., and Gale, A. (1999). Developing the role of the generic healthcare support worker: phase 1 of an action research study. *International Journal of Nursing Studies*, 36, 323–334.

Royal College of Nursing Policy Unit. (2009). The Assistant Practitioner Role: A Policy Discussion Paper, Policy Briefing 06/2009. London: Royal College of Nursing.

Royal Liverpool Children's Inquiry. (2001). The Royal Liverpool Children's Inquiry Report. www.gov.uk/government/publications/the-royal-liverpool-childrens-inquir y-report

Shakesby, A. and Wallace, C. (2012). Domestic violence: Top tips for support worker practice in Wales. *British Journal of Healthcare Assistants*, 6, 17–23.

Skills for Health. (n.d.). The Care Certificate. www.skillsforhealth.org.uk/standards/ item/216-the-care-certificate

Skills for Health. (2011). The Role of Assistant Practitioner in the NHS: Factors Affecting Evolution and Development of the Role. Bristol: Skills for Health.

Skills for Care and Skills for Health. (2013). Code of Conduct for Healthcare Support Workers and Adult Social Care Workers in England. www.skillsforhealth.org.uk/ standards/item/216-the-care-certificate

4 Knowing the law to keep ourselves and our clients safe

Paul Mackreth

Introduction

If you are reading this handbook from cover to cover, you have so far read and learned to appreciate how your work role and personal self are closely aligned in providing quality care. This chapter now moves on to the duties and responsibilities that are placed upon us by the law.

As you would have seen in the other chapters, there is a lot from our personal self that we bring into our job. Our first duty is as a member of the public, and it is our responsibility to comply with the law expected by the society in which we live. If you have not done so, then it is likely that you will be barred from being employed as a support worker. In some cases, you will be allowed to work, but we guarantee that there would have been some debate at your selection interview as to your suitability to work with vulnerable people as a support worker.

If you have picked up this book and come directly to this chapter (as many people do when reading a textbook!), then you are here to understand the law better. You may be concerned about something in practice that you have observed. If this is the case, then you will need to talk to someone and take some confidential advice without delay. This chapter is only an introduction to systems of the law. It is not a legal textbook. As you will see, laws are modified over time, and, therefore, on any question about the legality of practice or what may or may not be within the law more generally, you must seek advice as soon as possible. We can recommend the following sources, but please note that the contact numbers and the names of supportive organisations also change over time:

- NHS and Social Care Whistleblowing Helpline: 08000 724 725
- Citizens Advice (anyone can access)
- Safeguarding lead (NHS, social care and third sector)
- Duty of candour guardians (NHS)
- Care Quality Commission (CQC disclosure helpline: 03000 616161)
- Consultation with a solicitor or legal advisor (either by yourself or through your trade union affiliation or through independent organisations such as the charity Protect: 020 7404 6609).

As you will see from this chapter, the law in the UK is complex and does not just mean the law as put in place by the government. The law can be much more subtle as it can relate to what is expected of you at the time you practise. We do not wish to concern you, but you can be called to account for your practice many years after an event. Therefore, issues relating to how you communicate and keep records (as explored in Chapter 6) are very important.

Box 4.1 Activity: How were people cared for in the past?

Think about how people used to be cared for in the past. Let's say 50–100 years ago. Write down the things that you think were 'the norm' then, but are frowned upon or defined as illegal today. Now think about why this practice changed and what events led up to that change.

For example, tying someone to the bed 'for their own safety' was practised in the 1930s and became routine, but we know this 'routine' to be fundamentally wrong, and now it is categorised as physical abuse. The Mental Capacity Act (2005) and the Criminal Justice and Immigration Act (2008) have very strict conditions for when, how and in whose interest any form of restraint can be used.

Learning outcomes

At the end of this chapter you will be able to:

- Describe your duty to comply with the law in your personal life and how this can affect your role in support work
- Detail how the law is made in the UK
- Compare the different sources of information that you use to ensure that you are compliant with the law
- Articulate to others where to get help and advice.

Setting the scene

As indicated in the introduction to this chapter, we all have a duty to follow the law. Laws are often a measure of how fair, just and safe we are in our communities and wider society. We may not like some of these laws – for example, when the police started to enforce traffic laws, people often wondered why they were not 'out catching real criminals' – yet we all know that we need traffic laws to keep us safe.

In support work, our past personal life is open to checks through the Disclosure and Barring Service (DBS). Often, this is undertaken as an enhanced check that reports 'spent' convictions. These could be offences committed when someone was younger, when they received a police caution. If this is the case, then employers make a judgement about someone's suitability to work in a supportive and caring role. In our experience, this is often looked at pragmatically; for example, a shoplifting caution from 30 years ago when someone was a child is very different to having been cautioned for hitting someone, however long ago.

There is one overruling issue to consider in support work and the law. That is the duty, responsibility and accountability to protect the public. This duty is yours, your employer's and the government's. Remember 'the context' discussed in the previous chapter? The context of the law is very relevant to our practice. Over the years, we have seen lots of high-profile abuse cases. These have led the government, employers and workers to change practice, either through reflecting on roles or through a fundamental change in the law.

> ### Box 4.2 Care worker abuse
>
> Go to your internet search engine. Search 'care worker abuse'. Warning: what you will see is shocking and upsetting. You will often see how changes are suggested as the result of a conviction.

Look at your activity about what used to be legal that may not be now. What changed? When it comes to society, the context changes all the time; it shifts in what we hope is a progression towards a fairer, more just way of living. We no longer send children out to work for 12 hours a day, as people started to realise that this was wrong. Groups came together and asked Parliament to change the law, and this law continued to change to the point we are now where there is a right to be a child (Convention on the Rights of the Child, UN General Assembly 1989, and the Children Act, 2004).

Likewise, in care work, we now realise that people who need our help, support and care are incredibly vulnerable. There are now a whole host of laws in place to protect these vulnerable people. Laws will change over time, and so it is important that you keep up to date. For this reason we are not going to list all of the laws as they are subject to change and amendment. What we are doing is listing areas that are relevant to your support worker role at the time of writing. We hope that you will consider them and reflected upon them and see them as relevant to your practice.

How law is made in the UK

Statute

The most obvious method of law-making in the UK is based upon the government making laws through the Houses of Parliament. Your elected member of parliament (MP) will vote through, object to or seek amendments to bills presented initially to the House of Commons, either by the government or by individual MPs. Bills that pass through the House of Commons (MPs) and the House of Lords (appointed peers) and then receive royal assent from the queen become enacted as laws through the statute of Parliament.

The UK Houses of Parliament have a very good resource page where you can read about each of the stages, from MPs making a proposal (a draft bill) all the way through to becoming an Act of Parliament. See www.parliment.uk

This website also takes you to links where you can view all of the UK Acts. It also details how Acts are published, enacted, reviewed (post-legislative scrutiny) and even repealed. We suggest that you visit this website, as it is good to understand the foundations of our democratic process. We are very lucky to live in a country where we have a democratic process that is open, accessible and transparent.

If you want to explore democracy further, you can ask to meet your MP at their 'surgery'. Your local MP may use a local constituency venue or their constituency office to hold this surgery. You can take matters that concern you and talk them over. Your MP will be thinking about what legislation your issue falls under and if it is possible to amend or change it, or even try to detail for you why particular legislation is written in a certain way.

You can find details of your local MP by going to www.parliament.uk/mp s-lords-and-offices/mps/. This will also tell you how to contact them or follow them on social media.

If you ever want to visit the Houses of Parliament (the Palace of Westminster), then you can join a tour, watch a debate, attend a talk or even ask your MP for a guided tour! All of this is to ensure that you are engaged in the democratic process and that our process of making laws is open, honest and transparent.

Box 4.3 Example of how statute laws change over time

The Care Act (2014): see www.legislation.gov.uk/ukpga/2014/23/contents:

An Act to make provision to reform the law relating to care and support for adults and the law relating to support for carers; to make provision about safeguarding adults from abuse or neglect; to make provision about care standards; to establish and make provision about Health Education England; to establish and make provision about the Health Research Authority; to make provision about integrating care and support with health services; and for connected purposes.

This Act became law, but has been amended in a number of places; see the lengthy page on what changes are made in post-legislative scrutiny: www.gov.uk/government/publications/care-act-statutory-guidance/lis t-of-changes-made-to-the-care-act-guidance

---

Common law

However well laws are written, there is always an issue of interpretation of the law. The UK Parliament only enacts laws; it does not enforce them. This falls to other state institutions. Frequently, laws are tested in the courts, and decisions are made. Once a legal judgment has been made, it becomes a 'legal precedent'.

UK law is also based upon 'common law'. This is very different to statute law that remains on the statute books until it is repealed. Common law is when the facts of a case are brought to a judge to consider what is right or wrong. His or her verdict sets a precedent and, therefore, becomes common law. It makes the law of the UK very complicated and changeable over a short space of time. It is why we often need solicitors to guide us through the legal system, as they are skilled as looking at cases to find what is the most up-to-date legal precedent. This can be used to argue a case.

It should not be forgotten that this is further complicated by the geographical areas in which these decisions are made. Common law refers to the law being common to all. However, this is different in England and Wales (Courts of England and Wales) and may not refer to the judiciary of Scotland or Northern Ireland, who have a slightly different legal system – they have a separate judiciary (see below).

There is also the hierarchy of the legal decisions. A magistrate sits in a magistrates' court and does not have the power of precedent. It was thought that this would make laws too local. Criminal county courts do have this power, but these decisions can be challenged through the high courts – that is, the Court of Appeal or the Supreme Court.

Box 4.4 A case example: *Department for Education (DfE) v Jon Platt*

Jon Platt's case is a very good example of legal precedent and the hierarchy of courts in England (the information below is taken from and adapted from Long and Bolton 2017).

Section 444 of the Education Act 1996 states that children are required to attend school and that a fine may be given to parents if a child fails to attend 'regularly'. Jon Platt did not pay his fine as he argued successfully to a magistrates' court that his family holiday in school term time could not be defined as 'failing to attend regularly'.

As this was a magistrates' court, there was no legal precedent under common law. It may have been that Mr Platt had won, and no fine had to be paid, but his local authority was not content and, therefore, appealed their case to the next level of court, the High Court. The High Court upheld the magistrates' court's finding in favour of Mr Platt.

The Department for Education then went on to support the local authority in appealing the High Court decision to the Supreme Court. This, the highest court in England, found Mr Platt guilty, ordered him to pay £2,020 and gave him a 12-month conditional discharge.

This Supreme Court ruling means that we now have greater clarity over who can decide what constitutes school absence.

Devolved powers and different judiciary

As we can see, the law is a very complex area. It is more complex owing to the different judiciaries of Great Britain and Northern Ireland (the UK). Scotland and Northern Ireland have always had different judiciaries – for example, there are no magistrates' or criminal courts in Scotland, but in place they have sheriff courts, sheriff appeal courts and then a high court. Since the late 1990s (and updated more recently, in 2017 and 2018), Scotland, Wales and Northern Ireland have had devolved (or transferred – the term used in Northern Ireland) powers. Importantly for this textbook, these involve all aspects of health and social services.

Other areas of responsibility for the devolved or transferred powers are areas that can affect health, such as housing, education and benefits.

Devolution

Devolved powers mean that there are lots of different rules, processes, terminology and organisational names for health and social care (www.gov.uk/topic/government/devolution). One very good example of this are the different rules for holding and registering powers of attorney, where you ask someone to act in your interest if you no longer have the capacity to make decisions or can manage your day-to-day affairs. The different judiciaries are very different, and so, in England and Wales there are 'lasting' and 'ordinary' powers of attorney; Scotland uses 'continuing', 'welfare' or 'combined' powers of attorney; and Northern Ireland uses, 'enduring' or 'general' powers of attorney.

This is important as, if you move workplace to a different part of the UK, then you will start to see very different language, terms, laws and legal processes. It will be helpful for you to get to know the differences, why they are different and how your practice needs to differ.

Box 4.5 Activity: How different are codes of conduct in different countries?

Each of the four countries that make up our United Kingdom have their own code of conduct. This is because each country has its own devolved/transferred powers when it comes to matters of health and social care. A question arises, therefore: how different is each of these codes of conduct?

Have a look at each of them and work out how different they are. For example, in Northern Ireland, the code is only referred to as being for 'social care'.

Europe

Over the last few decades, Europe has had a significant impact upon UK laws. Although the UK has the Supreme Court as the highest authority, the UK also recognises that European Union laws have 'supremacy' and, therefore, relate to

UK law. This has allowed people to seek a higher judgment from the EU Courts of Justice if they felt that EU Law was not adhered to. This has allowed them to obtain a judgment where recommendations might be made to UK policy.

EU law has been fundamental to the UK's developing or adopting legislation to ensure that it continues to have parity with European legislation. One very good example of this is the European Working Time Directive on working conditions (www.fullfact.org). This will directly impact on your role as a support worker and offer you significant protection in your work.

It is also important to point out that, whatever the outcome of Brexit, the impact of EU law upon all parts of UK legislation is and will continue to be profound. Depending upon the deal between the UK and the EU, it may be likely that we are subject to these EU laws for some time. EU courts may still be referred to for anything that has occurred before the date on which the UK leaves the EU.

In writing this handbook, we have attempted to find examples of how EU laws impact upon our roles. What we found is that there is a very confused picture, with lots of mixed messages and suggested 'fake news'. We presume that this has occurred given the passion people have felt in the Brexit debate, but it is very unhelpful when seeking up-to-date, accurate information.

What we have found is that there are some very good resources available to find the 'truth behind the rumours', and we can recommend the Full Fact (www.fullfact.org) web resource as a way of deciding if and how EU law has determined our structures for support workers' and other health workers' practice.

Standards of care underpinned by the law

Every aspect of our care is expected to be to a high standard – our 'duty of care' is underpinned by a variety of laws that set out these expectations (Griffith 2014). This is about what you do, what you do not do (omission) and how you communicate and advise people. These are often referred to as standards of care. They are most notable in professional or medical practice where there may be high levels of risk and liability – for example, in medical surgery – but affect each and every aspect of our practice.

If a case were brought by a claimant, you would have to defend what you did or did not do against the standard of care expected for when you practised. These standards may be based upon the 'evidence base' at the time or underpinned by state law such as the Equality Act (2010) or the Mental Capacity Act (2005). In legal terms, this becomes 'the instrument'. It is also likely to be what the expectation of practice was on the day in question.

A famous case from common law that established this was *Bolam v Friern Hospital Management Committee*. Mr Bolam consented to have electro-convulsive therapy that, when administered, caused him to have such a large seizure that he was injured. Mr Bolam argued that he should have been made aware of the risks and given muscle relaxants to prevent the severity of his seizure.

The hospital successfully argued in court that this was not the standard of practice, and, therefore, there was no neglect. This is now referred to as the Bolam Test (Griffith 2014). It has been modified since the case, and there are many other tests and instruments to ascertain standards of care and practice.

However, the message to learn from this is that we must follow all the standards expected of us. This becomes our legal duty of care. This also involves where we decide not to do something.

Box 4.6 Discussion point

Support worker codes of conduct are not very well known. Yet they clearly set out standards and expectations for practice. How well do you and your employer know them, and could they be used as part of a Bolam Test?

Conclusion

We set out in this chapter to provide you with an overview of some of the legal processes in the UK. You will see that they are complex and varied. We hope that you agree that it is helpful to understand some of the broader principles of how law is made and adapts. The result of this is that you must always seek advice from other professionals and services who can support you.

Laws have been put in place to protect the public and our clients, who can be vulnerable members of society. Their legal protection will continue to be strengthened, sometimes thanks to the whistleblowing or advocacy of others.

The law places a huge burden upon us as healthcare workers, regardless of our role. We must follow the standards of care expected and raise concerns where this is not happening. To this end, we offer important contacts on the opening page of this chapter.

Laws – for example, health and safety legislation – are also there to protect us and our health, and so it is incumbent on us to work with them to protect ourselves and the health of our colleagues.

In the longer term, we hope that you will engage in the democratic process, use the resources above to get to know the parliamentary process and even go and meet your MP to discuss matters of your work with them. Only through this process can we see longer-term change that will continue to allow our clients to live to their potential.

Box 4.7 Further activity: Follow-up reading

We expect that many of you will have annual statutory and mandatory training to ensure that you are aware of many of the laws that direct how you go about working as a support worker, but, to ensure that you are aware of your responsibilities, you may want to follow this up with reading on the following legislation:

- Equality and diversity
- Health and safety
- Safeguarding adults and children
- Data protection
- Mental capacity.

References

Care Act (c 23). (2014). London: HMSO.

Children Act (c 31). (2004). London: HMSO.

Criminal Justice and Immigration Act (c 4). (2008). London: HMSO.

Equality Act (c 15). (2010). London: HMSO.

Griffith, R. (2014). Duty of care is underpinned by a range of obligations. *British Journal of Nursing*, 23(4), 234–235.

Long, R. and Bolton, P. (2017,19 April). Briefing paper: Holidays during school term-time (England). House of Commons Library, no 07590.

Mental Capacity Act (c 9). (2005). London: HMSO.

UN General Assembly. (1989, 20 November). Convention on the Rights of the Child, United Nations, Treaty Series, vol. 1577, p. 3. Available at: www.refworld.org/docid/3ae6b38f0.html (accessed 29 June 2020).

5 Knowing how to be with people

Bryony Walker

Introduction

This chapter has a strong relationship to Chapter 2, 'Knowing yourself', so, if you have forgotten Chapter 2 or have skipped it, we do suggest you go back and read it. We want you to move from appreciating the value and importance of self-awareness in support work to being able to see how, as a 'self-aware' support worker, you can then focus on the all-important relationship between yourself and the patients/clients/service users you work with. We will introduce you to the frequently used phrase 'person-centred care' and discuss some of the challenges that can be presented to the support worker in practice. We will start to unpick some of the language that is frequently used under the umbrella concept of person-centred care and use scenario examples to enable you to think about your own decision making. We will also discuss some of the communication skills that can help build the patient–client relationship.

Learning outcomes

At the end of this chapter you will be able to:

- Understand the meaning of 'person-centred care' and how central the support worker role is to its effective delivery
- Identify when barriers or challenges to person-centred care present themselves in your practice area
- Discuss the qualities and skills required for active listening in person-centred care

Setting the scene

The Cavendish Report, published in 2013, was very clear that you, the support worker, are the practitioner most likely to spend the most time by the bedside of the patient in hospital. Stonehouse (2014, p. 397), in his article discussing the importance of communication skills in the support worker role, also concluded, 'Support workers are ideally placed to support and facilitate good quality communication in the workplace'. In order to be able to do this, the support worker needs to be equipped with the skills to be able to build the relationship. Wherever you work in the UK, if your work is informed by a code of conduct, you will be expected to respect the privacy, confidentiality and dignity of the people you work with and communicate effectively with them and all those involved in their care. The skills required by the support worker to be person-centred in the relationship with the clients and their families can go unrecognised in the busy world of health and social care; however, the evidence is that they can contribute to the speed of the patient's recovery.

Person-centred care

Person-centred care does literally mean putting the person at the centre of their care. The phrase can be found in countless policy documents and is referred to by the various health and social care professional bodies and on their registration websites. In 2016, the Health Foundation broke it down into the following four principles:

1. Affording people dignity, compassion and respect.
2. Offering coordinated care, support or treatment.
3. Offering personalised care, support or treatment.
4. Supporting people to recognise and develop their own strengths and abilities to enable them to live an independent and fulfilling life.

(Health Foundation 2016, p. 7)

However, as you will have started to appreciate from earlier examples, being consistently person-centred in practice is a tough goal for care providers to achieve for countless reasons. In light of the four principles above, support workers can often feel that they hold responsibility for a very small part of the 'person-centred care' being delivered. It is the view of the authors that the central skill of the support worker is the responsibility for building the relationship with the patient and their family. Relationship building and effective communication are extremely important responsibilities in health and social care.

As a result of several high-profile cases raising serious concerns about the standards of care provided to patients within the NHS, the Six Cs of nursing were introduced in 2012. An NHS commission consulted with patients and service users, and, although some of you reading this book will not be part of NHS services or linked directly to nursing care, the values found have impacted on the worlds of both and health and social care, and so some of the language used can be found in support worker code-of-practice documentation. Below are the Six Cs statements from the Compassion in Practice policy document. Please read and attempt to answer the following questions, notice where the gaps in your knowledge are and take action to resolve this.

Box 5.1 Reflective activity using the Six Cs (Department of Health 2012, p. 13)

Care

Care is our core business and that of our organisations, and the care we deliver helps the individual person and improves the health of the whole community. Caring defines us and our work. People receiving care expect it to be right for them, consistently, throughout every stage of their life.

Task: If you are working in an organisation now, please write down three things you notice about the place where you work that communicates the above statement clearly to your patient/client group and their families and carers.

Compassion

Compassion is how care is given through relationships based on empathy, respect and dignity – it can also be described as intelligent kindness and is central to how people perceive their care.

Task: Reflect on your last act of 'intelligent kindness' with a patient or client.

Competence

Competence means all those in caring roles must have the ability to under-stand an individual's health and social needs and the expertise, clinical and technical knowledge to deliver effective care and treatments based on research and evidence.

Task: After reading this C statement, how competent do you feel in your support worker role today?

Communication

Communication is central to successful caring relationships and to effective team working. Listening is as important as what we say and do and essential for 'no decision about me without me'. Communication is the key to a good workplace with benefits for those in our care and staff alike.

Task: How well listened to do you feel in your current role?

Courage

Courage enables us to do the right thing for the people we care for, to speak up when we have concerns and to have the personal strength and vision to innovate and to embrace new ways of working.

Task: Do you know how to escalate concerns in your organisation?

Commitment

A commitment to our patients and populations is a cornerstone of what we do. We need to build on our commitment to improve the care and experience of our patients, to take action to make this vision and strategy a reality for all and meet the health, care and support challenges ahead.

Task: What activities have you been involved in as a support worker that demonstrate your commitment to improving the care and experience of the people you work with?

The Six Cs and your support worker code of conduct are excellent reminders of the values and standards patients and their families should expect us to uphold. However, patients can only experience the Six Cs within the relationship they have with you and other practitioners involved in their care.

The patient relationship starts with 'hello'

'Hello my name is' is a powerful social movement (www.hellomynameis. org.uk/), now global in impact, started by the late Dr Kate Granger who was diagnosed with terminal cancer and receiving treatment. Dr Granger noticed that, when she was a patient receiving care, health staff were not even bothering to introduce themselves before administering treatment, and so she started the 'Hello my name is ...' campaign. The core message of the campaign was to urge staff working in health and social care to, at the very least, introduce themselves to their patients at the start of the helping relationship. She firmly believed this would start a relationship that would then be capable of compassion. Her experiences gave her four values, detailed below. We think you will agree they are succinct and powerful and also come at very low cost to the practitioner or service. Dr Kate Granger died in 2016, but the website she and her husband developed is still available; it is inspirational and worth a look. The values are simple and easy for any practitioner to deliver.

Box 5.2 'Hello my name is ...'

- If you don't know the patient you are working with, ensure you introduce yourself to them.
- Remember 'the little things' when working with the patient as they do matter.
- Put the patient at the centre of everything.
- See the person before the patient.

Activity

- Can you think of an example where, when you were a patient, the practitioner did not introduce themselves to you?
- Think about some of 'little things.' Dr Kate Granger might be referring to here – for example, remembering how someone likes their tea.

(Source: Key values adopted by the 'Hello my name is …' campaign, www.hellomynameis.org.uk/key-values/)

Compassion

Dr Granger's message is clear: by introducing ourselves to the patient we signal to them that we, the practitioners, intend to build a connection that will support the growth of compassion. In Chapter 2, compassion fatigue was mentioned as something you must be aware of. The concept of compassion has many definitions, but the one that follows works for the helping relationship:

> the sensitivity shown in order to understand another person's suffering, combined with a willingness to help and to promote the wellbeing of that person, in order to find a solution to their situation.
>
> (Perez-Bret, Altisent and Rocafort 2016, p. 599)

Box 5.3 The 'I' test

Think of the last time someone showed you compassion.

- What did they say?
- How did they behave towards you?

Compassion and care go hand in hand and keep the person at the centre. We hope that earlier chapters of this book have perhaps supported you to reflect on the possibility that you might have 'unknown' spots (see Johari's window) that mean you could be challenged by circumstances or patients that, therefore, test your ability to demonstrate compassion. In health and social care, it is entirely possible at times, owing to time restrictions and limited resources, to base our roles and responsibilities around the tasks we are expected to do for or with our patients. We can even do these tasks without noticing who the person in front of us is. For example, we can ask people to roll over so that we can change their bedsheets, ask them what they want to put on their shopping list or even take them to the surgery and leave them without acknowledging how they are or even who they are. Families and carers can also get the same treatment: we might say hello to them, but then turn our attention to getting the task done. We can justify this to ourselves by thinking we are not inter-fering. However, we are there, in the room, and so they do see us.

> ## Box 5.4 Scenario: Lillian
>
> Jill is a care worker for Lillian, who is in her 90s. She helps her to get up and prepares breakfast for her every day. Jill has done this for the last 18 months. Today, as she helps her transfer out of bed, Lillian winces in pain. Jill does notice but, fearing she would be late for her next visit, pretends that she does not notice.
>   What is Jill more concerned with here?

Jill's compassion has been reduced as she feels the pressure of time. Lillian is no longer the person at the centre of the care: her pain is being overlooked in favour of Jill's schedule. Time is now at the centre, and Jill is not seeing things from her patient's point of view.

Barriers to person-centred care for the patient

Person-centred care isn't complex to comprehend, but can be very challenging to deliver, and there can be obstacles and barriers that might be nothing that you, the support worker, have any control over. In their study, Lloyd, Elkins and Innes (2018) identified staffing constraints, poor staff attitudes, high work-loads and time pressures, and poor resources, and the list goes on.

> ## Box 5.5 Activity: Barriers to person-centred care
>
> - Can you identify any barriers to person-centred care in your own work environment?
> - What are the consequences for the people you work with?

> ## Box 5.6 Activity: Ava
>
> ### Scenario
>
> Ava is 86 years old and has been diagnosed with vascular dementia. She is now living in a care home that claims to specialise in dementia. Ava's hus-band died of cancer more than 20 years ago, and they did not have any children. Before her illness became too advanced, Ava used lasting powers of attorney to appoint one friend her property and financial affairs attorney and another friend her health and welfare attorney. Both parties are invited to the care home one day and told that the care home, which describes

itself as being able to care for people with advanced dementia, can no longer 'handle' Ava's behaviour, which is agitated. The friends are given mixed messages by staff, but no real explanation is provided. They are given a week to find a new place for Ava to live. Ava's friends have been left feeling that, now the care home has made the decision, even if they appeal, Ava will be at risk of a poor standard of care.

Activity

Look back at the Six Cs. What would have been the person-centred approach here for Ava and her friends?

Promoting dignity

'Dignity' is quite difficult to define until we know that it has been lost or taken away from us. It can often be used to replace 'embarrassment' or 'humiliation' or something we have experienced that we now feel ashamed of. 'I lost my dignity.' It can even happen when we trip over in the street: although we are unhurt, we are left feeling as though we did not represent ourselves well, and, if a couple of people witnessed the fall, it might add to the feelings of 'loss of dignity'. Our sense of dignity can also be connected to our age, gender, sexual orientation, ability/disability, culture, ethnicity, religion – the list goes on.

For example, if a young child falls in the street, the child will probably focus more on the shock of the fall than the feeling of humiliation of doing so in front of a small crowd, whereas a person in their 30s might notice those around them more than the injury. In healthcare and social care, we provide intimate care, and this can mean that maintaining a person's dignity is always in the balance alongside the kind of care we need to offer to maintain safety, hygiene and nutritional needs.

Box 5.7 Common core principles to support dignity in adult social care services

- Value the uniqueness of every individual
- Uphold the responsibility to shape care and support services around each individual
- Value communicating with individuals in ways that are meaningful to them
- Recognise and respect how an individual's dignity may be affected when supported with their personal care
- Recognise that an individual's surroundings and environments are important to their sense of dignity
- Value workplace cultures that actively promote the dignity of everybody
- Recognise the need to challenge care that may reduce the dignity of the individual.(Source: https://ccpdignity.co.uk/)

> **Box 5.8 Activity: Scenario – Peter**
>
> Peter, who is 80 years old, is on the ward recovering from a stroke. He is disorientated and confused at the moment. He has had a bed wash, but someone has left him without a sheet, and he is now naked in view of the rest of the people on the ward. You have noticed this.
>
> *Reflective question*
>
> What would be your next step to provide Peter with dignified care?

I suppose the first question to address is, if you were Peter, what would you want? Clearly, it is not culturally acceptable to be naked in public, and so maybe the answer is straightforward: you would cover Peter with a sheet and maybe draw the curtains round his bed.

The Dignity in Care Campaign (www.dignityincare.org.uk/About/) was set up in response to public concerns about the dignity of older people in care. Box 5.9 has its ten-point dignity challenges for services to achieve in order to be offering high-quality care.

> **Box 5.9 The ten dignity dos**
>
> 1 Have a zero tolerance of all forms of abuse
> 2 Support people with the same respect you would want for yourself or a member of your family
> 3 Treat each person as an individual by offering a personalised service
> 4 Enable people to maintain the maximum possible level of independence, choice and control
> 5 Listen and support people to express their needs and wants
> 6 Respect people's right to privacy
> 7 Ensure people feel able to complain without fear of retribution
> 8 Engage with family members and carers as care partners
> 9 Assist people to maintain confidence and positive self-esteem
> 10 Act to alleviate people's loneliness and isolation
>   (www.dignityincare.org.uk/About/The_10_Point_Dignity_Challenge/)

Creating the right conditions for the relationship with the patient

As a support worker working with people from many different backgrounds, you will need to communicate in a way that builds trust in the people you work with. In the field of counselling, there is a very well-known seminal thinker called Carl Rogers. Rogers is known for having created a school of person-centred counselling that thrives today, and, yes, the phrase 'person-centred' does have its origin there. Rogers shared a lot of similar beliefs about human beings and how they thrive with Abraham Maslow, mentioned in Chapter 2. He believed that, in order for people to grow in a counselling relationship, they need to have the right conditions. He wrote a seminal article in 1957 called 'The Necessary and Sufficient Conditions of Therapeutic Personality Change' and is known for putting the client at the centre.

Core conditions

Congruence

Another word for this might be 'genuineness'. The support worker role can sometimes make us feel distant from those we work with. It is not always possible to agree with our patients and the decisions they make, but usually people respect a professional if they can see a genuineness or authenticity to their work with them. Patients will notice when you hurry them or address concerns that relate only to your agenda, but they will respond better if they notice you are authentic in your response to them.

Reflective exercise

How do you observe genuineness in the people in your life? It might be they listen well, without interrupting, and you can tell they have listened to you because they can detail the words and language you used as you were talking. They may also be open and honest if they don't know the answer to questions, but instil confidence that, even though they did not have the answer, they were clear they would find it out. They do this because they care and they take responsibility for the gaps in their knowledge. Because they do this, you can feel your confidence in your relationship with them grow.

Unconditional positive regard (UPR)

In your work, you will meet people who will test your patience and behave extraordinarily badly. Of course, none of us goes to work to be verbally or physically abused or assaulted, and appropriate and immediate action should be taken in these circumstances. However, some people you work with will, for complex reasons, have little or no self-worth and will have never experienced a positive relationship, and they only know how to lash out when they seek help. In these circumstances, the support worker has an opportunity to demonstrate acceptance, kindness and understanding in their actions toward these patients and clients. Taking a UPR approach can sometimes show to people in crisis and at their worst that they are still worth something. However, there are consequences.

Box 5.10 Scenario: Emily

Emily comes into A&E for the fourth time in 7 days, completely drunk again. She has now injured her hand, and it needs stitching. In her drunken state, she calls you a 'fat shit' in a busy waiting room. Her behaviour is challenging, and she is particularly focused on embarrassing you. She clearly needs care, and her behaviour is not so bad that you need to call the police.

Your feelings

You do not like this woman; she is making you uncomfortable and your patience is being tested. She also reminds you of someone you do not like, but you must offer her care.

- How would you approach Emily in order to provide her with compassionate care and demonstrate UPR?
- What steps would you take to make sure you are ok?

Empathy

The empathy versus sympathy debate is quite an active one in the field of the health and social care. The reality is that, as a support worker, you will experience both and offer both to the people you work with. However, genuine empathy will help you see things from the patient's perspective rather than your own, or, in the words of Carl Rogers (1957, p. 99), enable you 'to sense the client's private world as if it were your own'. In order to help people, you will have to walk in their shoes, and, although it is realistic to understand that the view from their shoes will be informed by who you are, working hard at empathy can help you build a positive relationship with a patient and it can also help you identify their resources and strengths, as well their needs.

Let's return to Emily. This time, you take an opportunity to talk to her, even though she is drunk and has been abusive.

Box 5.11 Emily

YOU: Emily, this is your fourth visit to A&E this week?
EMILY: It's not a bloody crime, is it?
YOU: I have just noticed that's all. What's going on?
EMILY: Social Services have taken my children. Fucking bastards!
YOU: So, you're upset and because of this you are hitting the bottle more?
EMILY: Yup.
YOU: That must be really tough for you.

In this scenario, the support worker does not get distracted by the combative response, but instead continues with reflecting back what they have noticed and showing an interest in Emily. The outcome of the brief exchange is that Emily gives the support worker an important piece of information that does, to an extent, provide an explanation for her behaviour. There is now a window of opportunity to support Emily more; it might also mean that she gets a more compassionate response, even though her behaviour is challenging.

Active listening skills

Listening to people is harder than we think. People are not always that interesting to be honest. You might be able to pinpoint examples from your own life where your head has been somewhere else and someone finally punctures your thoughts by shouting, 'You are not listening to me!' Obviously, when we have a natural rapport with someone, we listen, or, if they are telling us something we find riveting or important to us, that might be straightforward. Then, we do not need to consciously think to listen. When listening is a core part of your role, it is essential to understand the importance and skill of active listening if you are going to build a relationship with patients. Patients will notice (as they should) if you are not making the effort to listen to them, and this will impact on the quality of care you can deliver. From their perspective, you are disconnected, you do not truly see them, and, although they might have to co-operate with the care you offer, they will not provide you with much more information.

Below are some helpful active listening skills, taken from the field of counselling. These skills can take practice, and, when we teach these skills in the classroom, students sometimes report that the skills feel unnatural to them and make the conversation feel weird. However, students also report that, when they apply these skills in practice, they can see the benefits to the relationship.

Box 5.12 Example: Paraphrasing

PATIENT: It's been several days since I have fancied eating anything at all, just had a couple of bananas to settle tummy, but that is it.
YOU: You have had a few bananas in the last few days but not much else, am I correct?

Box 5.13 Example: Clarifying

YOU: Can I just ask you to clarify, how many days have you only managed to eat bananas?
PATIENT: I think it could be 4 days.
YOU: Oh, so quite a long time, then.

Box 5.14 Example: Reflecting

PATIENT: I don't think I am feeling myself after the anaesthetic, I am completely wiped and can't do anything.
YOU: You say you are wiped out since the anaesthetic? Must be tough for you, as you are usually a very active person, aren't you?

Box 5.15 Example: Summarising

YOU: So, let me see if I have listened to you. You say you are still feeling groggy after the operation. You have only had a few bananas to eat in the last few days. You are feeling wiped out. Have I missed anything important?
PATIENT: No, that's correct.

Body language or non-verbal communication

Imagine you are with a patient who is being given some very bad news. You are holding the hand of someone who is being told that their diagnosis will limit their life expectancy. Any decent human being understands that a yawn and phone check for messages from the support worker at this point would be entirely inappropriate, interpreted as callous even, and may lead to a reprimand and even the start of a disciplinary process if you are caught behaving that way more than once. If you wish to convey to patients that you are compassionate, empathetic and listening, you will have to think about your body or what is sometimes called non-verbal communication (NVC) language. It does not always come naturally to appear open for conversation and available for a chat.

Traditionally, it has been drilled into health and social care students that the way to connect with the patient is to ensure we position ourselves near to them, use open body language, which means not crossing our arms and legs, and make use of eye contact. However, body language and NVC do not always translate across different cultures. The traditional advice that we must always use eye contact works for most situations with many of our patients, but there might be exceptions to the rule. Using our bodies as 'language' can really help build rapport for some of our patients. When a patient suddenly clutches their arm and winces in pain, if we mirror the wince they showed us back to them, it can communicate that we have noticed what they are going through.

Touch and physical contact

Depending on the setting you work in, and the people you care for, there could be moments of physical contact, and some of this might be intimate care if you are working with vulnerable people such as the elderly or people who have a high degree of dependency on others because of disability or health conditions. You will support people to carry out daily living activities such as washing, dressing and using the toilet. It is important to remember that, throughout the human lifespan, these daily activities are usually carried out independently, except when we are infants or young children; therefore, another person – whether a health professional or a member of one's own family – helping in these areas can feel very challenging or disempowering for the person. Other factors can also interact with how a person might be challenged by support in intimate care, such as culture, ethnicity, religious belief, age – please add to the list if you can. Please ensure that you follow your organisation's policy and practice on intimate care. A very simple rule for touch is always to ask (gain consent) the person before you touch them in any way.

Touch is also used by humankind to connect with another person and for reassurance; as part of NVC, it can be very powerful and healing within the caring relationship. There are different types of touch. Two examples of touch (Karatay, Gürarslan, Dogan and Oruker 2020) are:

- Instrumental touch: for example, when you help someone transfer from their bed to a chair
- Expressive touch: for example, touching someone's arm to give them reassurance when they are telling you something that is upsetting them. This touch expresses warmth and kindness.

Box 5.16 Scenario: John

John has suffered a spinal cord injury and is now partially paralysed. He has only recently been transferred to the spinal injuries ward. He is 27 years old, has lived alone for the last 3 years and had a very full life. He is struggling to come to terms with his injury and is angry when nursing staff wash him. You are a nursing assistant who has been asked to assist.

- How might you prepare yourself to assist him?
- What can you do to enable John to feel he has some control?

In this chapter, you have been introduced to the principles of person-centred care and the importance of dignity. You have had some active listening skills to practise and, hopefully, with a growing self-awareness from the tools practice in

Chapter 2, you are starting to see how central your role is to the delivery of high-quality care to patients and their loved ones.

References

Karatay, G., Gürarslan, B. N., Dogan, S., and Oruker, M. (2020). Barriers of nursing students about touching: In general life and clinical settings. *International Journal of Caring Sciences*, 13(1), 675–682.

Perez-Bret, E., Altisent, R., and Rocafort, J. (2016). Definition of compassion in healthcare: A systematic literature review. *International Journal of Palliative Nursing*, 22 (12), 599–606.

Department of Health. (2012). Compassion in Practice Nursing Midwifery and Care Staff: Our Vision and Strategy. Commissioning Board Chief Nursing Officer and DH Chief Nursing Adviser.

Bradley, L., Mark, E., and Lesley, I. (2018). Barriers and enablers of patient and family centred care in an Australian acute care hospital: Perspectives of health managers. *Patient Experience Journal*, 5(3), 55–64.

The Health Foundation. (2016). *Person-Centred Care Made Simple*. London: The Health Foundation.

Lloyd, B., Elkins, M., and Innes, L. (2018). Barriers and enablers of patient and family centred care in an Australian acute care hospital: Perspectives of health managers. *Patient Experience Journal*, 5(3), 55–64.

Rogers, C.R. (1957). The necessary and sufficient conditions of therapeutic personality change. *Journal of Consulting Psychology*, 21(2), 95–103.

Stonehouse, D. (2014). Communication and the support worker. *British Journal of Healthcare Assistants*, 08(08), 394–397.

Skills for Care and Skills for Health. (2013). Code of Conduct for Healthcare Support Workers and Adult Social Care Workers in England. http:// tinyurl.com/ljr5dns

6 Knowing how to keep accurate records

Paul Mackreth

Introduction

The previous chapters in this book have been written to support your role, providing you with new information about your role and building a picture of what we consider is good support worker practice. This and subsequent chapters deal with more pragmatic issues in your practice, things that you can do to ensure that your client gets the best care and support and you feel rewarded by the work that you do.

This chapter is written specifically to remind you about your duty to record, write, maintain and keep safe your client records. Although there is a clear requirement in law for you to do so (see Chapter 4), there are other aspects of record keeping that are good practice, such as communicating with colleagues or providing a written narrative history about a person being cared for.

However, many people become aware of the importance of keeping good records through the worst scenario – being called upon to account for their actions. How do you do this? The answer is that you refer back to the records that you kept at the time. So, you need to ask yourself, what if I can't read them? What if I did not write down something that I did? How do I account for doing something if I did not write it down? Did I do it?

The other aspect of good record keeping is that others who you work with can see what has been undertaken, what you have observed and what is to happen next. Communication through good record keeping is vital to good and effective care and support.

Learning outcomes

At the end of this chapter you will be able to:

- Detail your duty and responsibility to maintain accurate records
- Describe some of the complications of writing records
- Compare your records with good practice criteria
- Make changes to your methods of record keeping, ensuring good practice and communication.

Each section that follows has a list of activities or directs you to other activities that you can undertake

Setting the scene

Have you ever had to use your written account of an event in a court hearing or formal investigation or to explain your actions? We hope not, but for some of you this may be a reality. The challenge of being held to account is why codes of conduct mandate that you 'maintain clear and accurate records of the healthcare, care and support you provide' (England, Skills for Care and Skills for Health 2013, n.p.); 'keep[ing] records that are up to date, complete, accurate and legible' (Northern Ireland, Northern Ireland Social Care Council, n.d., n.p.); and 'document and maintain clear and accurate records of your care' (Wales, GIG Cymru/NHS Wales, n.d., n.p.). NHS Scotland (2009) makes a number of different recommendations for record keeping in the Scottish code of conduct. All of these are to protect you and ultimately to protect the public.

The day job of support work practice is a busy place to work, and you need a good memory to get through your working day. So, how do you recall if you have done something or not? How do you recall if a client has given consent for care/support and/or intervention? How do you know if someone else has given a treatment? How do others around you know what has been done, what you observed, and what is left to do? We rely on written records for everything that we do.

Box 6.1 A short story on record keeping

Many years ago, Sam worked on a hospital ward. He recalls a client who had dementia and Sam felt uncomfortable about the ward environment, which was affecting the patient's mood and behaviour. Something just did not feel right. Was this the right place for him to be? Could his care needs be met, and would he come to harm if the ward environment was not adapted? As a registered nurse, Sam had responsibility to assess, plan, implement and evaluate the patient's care. In this instance, he knew that these records needed to be clear and precise and detail what had and had not been done. So, they were written in the knowledge that a good plan was needed, and that this might be scrutinized in future. He made sure that the care plan was specific to the patient's needs, and that anything recorded in it was not judgemental about the client's actions (which he could not control).

Many months later, he was called into the sister's office and asked to account for this client's ward experience. His family had questioned whether his care needs were met during his stay on the ward – they had also felt uncomfortable about his admission to hospital and the effect on his behaviour. Sam only had one thing to go on: the records kept at the time of the client's admission.

The short story in Box 6.1 shows that keeping good records helps to plan care, but also helps to recount care when needed. We should perhaps not be overly 'defensive' when keeping a record, but it is always a consideration and helps to explain to others many months after an event what we did, why we did it, and what plans we had. This is really the basis for open, honest and transparent care and, therefore, helps us in our 'duty of candour'. In this story, the records were used to communicate with family members what it was like for their loved one to stay on the ward. They detailed what was done and why. They were helpful in aiding the family to understand every aspect of the ward stay and what had been done to keep the environment safe.

Box 6.2 Activity: Your last set of records

Think about the last set of records that you wrote in (be honest) and consider the following:

- Can other people read them? Would they make sense?
- Are they in good chronological order?
- Do they properly set out what has been done and is left to do? Is the plan clear, unambiguous and up to date?
- Do they record the client's wishes and their consent for care?
- Are they written with good English grammar?

If the answer is yes to all the questions in Box 6.2, then you are moving in the right direction for keeping records. However, we suspect that for many readers the answer is no to one or more of these. What is offered in the following are some areas to work on.

Make sure you and others can read it and understand it accurately

Records are still frequently handwritten, particularly notes and records that are held by clients. When writing, we are often time-pressured, but *stop*, pause and think, 'Can I read this myself?' If you cannot, how can someone else?

Like any form of writing, records need to be clear and concise and have a purpose. You will often forget the purposes of record keeping that we detail above. Always have in the back of your mind that someone else *will* read this, either to understand what you have done or as a way of trying to communicate with colleagues.

A few tips for avoiding issues of not being able to read what has been written follow.

Abbreviations

Avoid abbreviations: health and social care are full of these. DNA (did not attend), MSU (mid-stream urine), TTO (to take home) – they plague our practice environment to the extent that a lay person would need a glossary of terms to understand our notes. So, what if someone were new to practice: would these help them understand what a client's needs were? We doubt it. If we are to look at good practice, let's avoid using them – DNU (do not use)!

> ### Box 6.3 Activity: The dangers of poor written communication
>
> The dangers of poor written communication in health and social care are well recorded. There are many examples of where this has led to harm. Paul recalls an incident when someone left a note saying, 'pregnancy test -ve, please phone to let them know'.
>
> Someone did make this phone call and informed the woman that she was pregnant. It was only later noticed that this abbreviation was intended to mean negative – that is, she was not pregnant. The person reading the note did not know the abbreviation and just saw the 've' and understood that to mean positive. They did not understand that the minus character before it meant 'negative'.

Colloquialisms

Colloquialisms are equally difficult. We live in the United Kingdom of Great Britain and Northern Ireland. Each country has its own language, dialect and accent. Although we are not suggesting a return to the Queen's English of the 1950s BBC, we suggest that you do not bring your 'regionality' into writing notes and records. So, if you practise in Northern Ireland, try to avoid writing that a client has 'boked' when vomited, or 'boaked' in Scotland, or 'chundered' in Lancashire. Paul remembers searching for a long time to find out what food a client had eaten, as a food diary suggested that a 'barm' had been eaten (a 'barm' is a bread bun, breadcake, bap, roll or butty).

Handwriting

It goes without saying that all handwriting should be legible (the convention is that it is also usually in black ink). All too often it is not. We joke about doctors' handwriting and laugh at how illegible it is. In reality, it is no laughing matter. If we want to communicate well, then we must put effort into how we write and write well. See the following for resources if this is an issue for you. Please also note that this is for any notes and phone messages, as well as the keeping of good client records.

The Irish National Adult Literacy Agency has a very good back-to-basics guide to improving handwriting. We recommend that you download a copy and work through it. It will mean printing a copy, and some of it may look very basic, but it is a nice exercise to work through. Note: Paul has done this and worked through it himself as his handwriting was awful; we like the section on choosing a pen (www.nala.ie/publications/handwriting-book/).

There are other guides to writing, and you may find other adult learning resources (such as www.cherrellavery.co.uk, featured by the *Daily Telegraph* and *The Guardian* newspapers).

Box 6.4 Activity: Typographical errors

Going back to the pregnancy test error above, the root cause analysis of the event found that the handwritten note was confusing: '-ve' was written very close to the 'P' for pregnancy and, at a glance, did indeed look like 'P-ve' – a hyphenated 'positive'.

Many drug chart and prescribing errors can be found to be down to abbreviations and/or poor handwriting. Even in electronic format, just look at the last few texts you have sent – how many of these have unintended meanings or typographical errors?

Order

Think about the order of what you have written. Does it make sense? Try to get a system to follow to guide this order. This will depend upon the records that you are writing, but handwritten notes don't often have headings, and so it is important. A blank white page is a very daunting thing to write on. A very popular tool for communicating is SBAR: situation, background, assessment and recommendations. SBAR is an increasingly popular tool to use to communicate in health settings (Blom, Petersson, Hagell and Westergren, 2015); it meets the demands of good record keeping in that it is clear, concise and specific. It steers you away from things that may be a matter of your own opinion (see later). In your role as a support worker, you may not be assessing and so you may want to adapt the tool and, in place of 'assessment', insert 'observation'.

Box 6.5 Activity: The SBAR acronym

Think of a client you have looked after (please do remember to maintain confidentiality) and consider how you have written up the notes for the next person to review the care given. Consider how you wrote these and how they may be made clearer by use of the SBAR acronym:

- Situation
- Background
- Assessment/observations
- Recommendations.

Only facts

The SBAR acronym also helps you to write facts only and not to be judgemental. How much and what to write should not be dictated by the time that you have, but by the facts as you have observed them. This is a very hard skill to master, as we all have a tendency to write emotion into facts. However, good records are factual and non-judgemental. Paul recalls reading a long record about how a client was:

> rude and not very nice to me and my colleague, he was so cross and used bad language, so we left and we called the nurse as we won't be talked to like that.

Although we don't want to belittle how it is hard to communicate with clients when they are agitated and come across as being aggressive, this was a very judgemental way to write up the notes. When Paul called to assess the client, he found the client was suffering from hypoxia, and this was the probable cause of his agitation and confusion. The more correct way to write this could have been:

S: On arrival we found Mr X acting agitated.

B: Mr X has chronic obstructive pulmonary disease (COPD) and is on continuous oxygen.

A: We observed Mr X for a few moments and were unable to communicate with him whilst he was agitated. He appeared very angry and we could not reason why.

R: A nurse visit is required to assess him.

Not repetitive

Records that are not repetitive are helpful for the reader of your notes and records. It goes without saying that reading the same thing over and over is not a good use of time. Records that repeat 'care as planned' may be a requirement from your employer to ensure that people know if you have delivered care, but pages and pages of the same record are largely unhelpful to find out what has been undertaken. It may be that small changes can be made to make them more meaningful or more significant. Could you consider making small observations? Again, SBAR may help with how concise and precise these are. For example, in a home care setting, these could be:

S: Mr X at home and sitting in his living room as expected.

B: Care package in place with no recommendations for changes to be made.

A: We observed Mr X was pleased to see us and looked forward to his lunch today. He drank a cup of tea and a glass of water when we were present.

R: No new recommendations.

Up to date and in the moment

Our final tip is to make sure that all records and notes are up to date and in the moment. This is very important to ensure all information is contemporary, but also that you do not add notes to records after an event.

We recall that there was once a time when we worked on a shift and then, towards the end of the shift, we would write up all the client records. This was bad practice and would not meet the standards of today's practice. First, records should be up to date for anyone who wants or needs to read them. It therefore follows that records should be updated as soon as possible after an event – that is, the delivery of care or support. If you do have to update records at a later date, then these records should indicate that they were updated at a later date. Be open and honest and never falsify information, such as the date that the information was written up.

It may be that you don't feel that you have time. You may find that many clients are happy for you to take time to write up the records. It will just need working into the conversation with them – for example, 'I need 5 minutes to write these up, is that okay?'

Link to organisational guidance and training

Your own employer, particularly a larger organisation, will have specific training for you to undertake to ensure that all staff are up to date with record keeping. Have you undertaken this training? We often find that training helps in the short term, but then the bad habits of record keeping creep back in.

You will notice that employer training also focuses upon how to keep records safe and confidential. The Data Protection Act (2018) and, within this, the General Data Protection Regulations (GDPR) place specific duties upon your employer (often the data controller) to look after the data for clients. As a data user/handler, you are also obliged to follow specific rules – do you know what these are? Do you know where to go if something goes wrong – for example, you lose some records or share information that you should not have?

Box 6.6 Activity: Data protection/record keeping

When writing and sharing information about clients, you should identify the following:

- When did you last do record keeping and/or data protection training?
- Who is the named person for information governance?
- Who is the data controller?
- Who are the data users/handlers?

We urge you to ensure that you know all of the answers to the questions in Box 6.6 as there are now very strict rules on how we handle records that inevitably contain personal information. This also includes what we can and cannot do with the information, based on consent and our legal duty.

Written or computer records

We have focused much of this chapter on the written record. Increasingly, records are electronic and not handwritten. There are many obvious advantages to this: for example, this ensures that they are accessible and can't be lost, they can be archived, don't have issues of legibility and tend to be very systematic. However, we also need to understand other factors. Sometimes, these systems can be complicated and require additional training. People need rights of access and permissions to use certain parts of computer systems. It can be hard to find where people have updated records, or, if you are not connected to the internet, some systems may not work at all.

Despite the challenges, there will inevitably be a move towards all records being kept electronically. So, the implications for your role are to ensure that you are up to date with your own IT skills and understand the terminology and how systems work; for example, when you log into a system it keeps a 'stamp' of what time you logged in, where in the system you have been and what you have written. This can be used to understand where you are if you work alone.

Data handling

Regardless of whether data are on a computer or tablet or in a written file, you must consider how and where these are kept and transported and what is expected in terms of access. Much of this relates to the expectations in GDPR detailed before, so do ensure that you are up to date and have sought guidance. You employer should have a very clear policy on this that you must ensure that you follow.

You must never be careless in relation to handling personal and sensitive information. If it is electronic, is it password-protected if your device was lost or taken? It needs to be. Where do you log on to the internet? Is it safe, or can people look over your shoulder at what you are typing?

If the information is in written form, who can see it if it's on your desk? Are you in a public place? Make sure it is secure, covered or kept in a file.

Transportation of information can be a huge issue. For paper files and electronic devices, this may involve being posted or emailed. Is it in your car? Should it be?

Good practice: Life stories and dementia

It may appear a little odd, but our example of good practice goes against some of the advice we have given earlier. In the search for advice on how to keep good records, we revisited the concept of 'life stories' (Andersson, Dellkvist, Johansson and Skär 2019). These are background stories that can be written to help those caring for people with dementia understand the person being cared for. Andersson et al. (2019) write that these can often be completed by close family members, help staff (in their case, care home staff) understand moral values and personal needs and detail significant life events of the person who has dementia. They can also help family members who write them feel a sense of purpose.

We recall one care home that did this very well. On meeting a client for the first time, we could see their life story in print and photographs and, therefore, understood the client as a person and not just as a person who is unwell with dementia and its symptoms. There was a photograph of this client on a cruise ship, and the life story detailed how she took to holidaying on cruise ships after she lost her husband. It listed the places she visited, friends that she met and the ships that she was on. It further detailed how this helped her deal with the loss of her husband.

It helped us to relate to the client and build an understanding of her as a whole person. The significance of this cannot be underestimated, as we noted the emotion it triggered in us and how it changed our attitude towards the client. It allowed us to see the client and not the illness.

The life story goes against some of the principles of SABR (which seeks to stop long storytelling) as it can be long and involve lots of emotion and detail, but the effect of having read this life story can really change how you approach someone in the attempt to be person-centered.

Conclusion

You will have learned that record keeping is a complex area where there are lots of areas for improvement. It is an area that we must continually revisit to ensure good practice and communication. It is also an area that can slip when we are most busy, and so, like other topics in this handbook, we must keep ourselves alert at all times.

We rely on records for lots of purposes and we all have a role to play in them. Not just the writing of them, but how they are written, communicated and transported. We must develop these skills to remain person-centered. Although there are times when records must be succinct, we have also learned that there are times when it is appropriate to have family members contribute to longer, more emotive life stories so that we can truly get to know clients as people and not just illnesses.

References

Andersson, E.K., Dellkvist, H., Johansson, U.B., and Skär, L. (2019). Relatives' experiences of sharing a written life story about a close family member with dementia who has moved to residential care: An interview study. *Nursing Open*, 6(2), 276–282.

Blom, L., Petersson, P., Hagell, P., and Westergren, A. (2015). The situation, background, assessment and recommendation (SBAR) model for communication between health care professionals: A clinical intervention pilot study. *International Journal of Caring Sciences*, 8(3), 530–535.

Data Protection Act (c 12). (2018). London: HMSO.

NHS Scotland. (2009). Code of Conduct for Healthcare Support Workers. The Scottish Government.

GIG Cymru/NHS Wales. (n.d.). Code of Conduct for Healthcare Support Workers in Wales. www.wales.nhs.uk/nhswalescodeofconductandcodeofpractice

Northern Ireland Social Care Council. (n.d.). Standards of Conduct and Practice for Social Care Workers. https://niscc.info/storage/resources/standards-of-conduct-and-practice-for-social-care-workers-2019-1.pdf

Skills for Care and Skills for Health. (2013). Code of Conduct for Healthcare Support Workers and Adult Social Care Workers in England. www.skillsforhealth.org.uk/standards/item/216-the-care-certificate

7 Know how to work in a person-centred way

Bryony Walker

Introduction

In Chapter 5, we looked at the some of the skills and 'ways of being' required to work in a person-centred way and how this will support us also to see the human being rather than just the medical condition or care needs we are working with. Health and social care services are designed to intervene in crisis and also to help people live with longer-term conditions. However, if you look at the NHS Long Term Plan (2019), the focus has shifted more and more to looking at how we can support people to live longer, healthier lives and have the tools to look after their own well-being. In a lot of health and social care literature, you will come across the words 'empowerment' and 'autonomy'. In this chapter, we will look at what these terms mean, but also consider some of the difficulties we can be faced with in practice when our patients or service users decide or wish to do things that we might view as 'risky' to their own health or well-being. We will also look at the some of the language of safeguarding and some of the challenges faced by those at risk of being stigmatised or overlooked because of their illness.

Learning outcomes

At the end of this chapter you will be able to:

- Understand the difference between person-centred and non-person-centred approaches
- Understand some of the challenges to working in a person-centred way
- Understand the importance of supporting choice, dignity and risk taking.

Setting the scene

In previous chapters, you have learned that the support worker should be equipped to understand the value of effective communication skills in order to help build relationships. You should work alongside the client/patient and view the whole person rather than just the care needs they have, noticing strengths and resources. At its best, the relationship between support worker and client is a collaborative partnership (Health Foundation 2016) that puts the patient/client at the centre of the decision making, which means seeing things from their perspective. The 'I' test below might help you to refocus on what it can be like to receive poor-quality care. In 2017, Kenward, Whiffin and Spalek published a research paper in the *British Journal of Nursing* that identified seven themes which emerged from several research papers on patients' views of feeling unsafe while using healthcare services. Please have a read through and see if you have experienced any of these concerns when you or a loved has received care.

Box 7.1 The 'I' test: Seven themes

Have you or a family member experienced the following when receiving treatment or care (adapted from Kenward et al. 2017)?

1 Information and communication: You did not get the information you needed about the care. There were changes made to care you were not involved in.
2 Loss of control: You were unable to move or talk. You could not look after you own self-care. Someone else made decisions on your behalf.
3 Staff presence: You could not find staff when you needed to. When staff were present, they were distracted. You were told to wait because staff had other things to attend to.
4 Impersonal care: Staff did not notice you as a unique person and did not, therefore, help you with the little things that are important only to you.
5 Vulnerable physical and emotional state: Staff did not notice how scared and anxious you were. They did not explain any of the routine to you and the medical devices you were using.
6 Not being taken seriously: When you made your needs known to staff, they did not act on them or take them seriously.
7 Perceived lack of staff experience: You were not convinced the staff caring for you were competent or had the appropriate training to look after you correctly.

From powerlessness to empowerment

Being a patient or needing support can be extremely unsettling physically, psychologically and socially, especially if you belong to a particularly vulnerable population of patients. Alistair Ross, an associate professor of psychotherapy at Oxford, wrote in 2016 of his experiences. He described returning to being a baby, again. He described being a patient as a time of 'radical helplessness' (2016, p. 275). Becoming a baby suggests he was reliant on others and incapable of looking after his own basic needs. Powerlessness is a common theme reported by patients, especially those where recovery is perhaps unclear or unlikely. Salomsé et al (2013) discuss the feelings of patients with leg ulcers and how their quality of life has been impacted in all areas.

If you look at the codes of practice for some of the professions you work with – for example, nurses, social workers, occupational therapists – you would find that they nearly all mention the word 'empowering'. The use of the word is usually connected to the profession expressing its commitment to support patients in setting goals and making informed decisions either about their treatment/care or their psychological and social needs. Empowering someone means enabling them to be active in their own decision making – for example, in their care or treatment plans. Empowering patients or carers can be easier said than done at times, especially if the clients you work with have long-term conditions or life-limiting conditions, as they might struggle to see the future. Empowerment can also be especially difficult to offer clients in a busy environment when resources are limited.

'Knowledge is power' is a common phrase, and your patients need knowledge in order to make their own decisions and to feel like they have some control, independence or – a commonly used word – autonomy in their lives. Depending on where you work, you will have responsibilities to ensure that the people you work with are (within their own capacity) aware of and involved in their treatment plans/care packages. You might not be the primary person responsible for conveying the information, but your role often puts you on the front line for questions, complaints, queries and so on, from both the patient and their family members. The key to a positive, empowering experience for the patient is how you respond.

Box 7.2 Example of a disempowering conversation

Oscar is a support worker for a mental health charity. He is visiting Adam, who has a diagnosis of psychosis and has just come out of hospital.

ADAM: My medication is really making me too tired to do anything. I want to play the guitar because it makes me feel better, but I can't concentrate, it is getting me down.

OSCAR: Adam, I understand as you keep mentioning this but as you know I am not able to change your medication. I am only a support worker and not your psychiatrist. You have an appointment in two weeks with your psychiatrist, so tell her then and she might change this.

Questions

- What is Oscar communicating to Adam?
- Where does the power lie?
- How would you feel if you were Adam in this scenario?
- How might you approach this situation differently and give Adam some choice, here, so that he doesn't feel so down?

Choice

Choice has been very briefly mentioned in the 'dignity dos' in Chapter 5, but what does it really look like in practice when we are in a helping relationship with the people we care for? If the patient is at the centre of everything we decide, then we need to be able to provide opportunities for choice. If we go to the GP with an illness and they prescribe medicine for us to take, a person-centred GP will tell us about the medication and discuss with us how long we need to take it, but they will also share the side effects or implications of taking the medication. It might be in our best interests to take the medication, but, as soon as we leave the GP surgery, we, the patient, will make the decision about whether we take the medication. We have the choice. The GP has made their best case to us, but, informed of the facts, we make the choice.

Choice can easily get washed away in our contact with patients; we can forget to offer them the time to process new information and hear the options. The tasks of the job can take over and dominate the time spent with patients, and then there is always the paperwork or clinical notes to get back to. Paperwork can loom large in our work routine and take us away from the valuable face-to-face time patients need from us to be well informed and involved in difficult decision making. Other work demands can also distract us and interrupt our ability to demonstrate the active listening skills discussed in Chapter 5, so please revisit if you need to review. Another challenge we can be faced with when we are listening to patient problems or challenges is that we can often feel their sense of powerlessness. In therapy, this would be called 'transference'. We might mirror this back to our patients. The support worker, Oscar, in the case above is essentially shrugging his shoulders and saying, 'C'mon Adam, live with it'. It might also be that Oscar feels powerless to support Adam to solve this issue; the difficulty is that Oscar's response lacks empathy, and he is forgetting how he would feel in Adam's shoes or if Adam was his son or brother.

Box 7.3 Here is the scenario again

ADAM: My medication is really making me too tired to do anything. I want to play the guitar because it makes me feel better, but I can't concentrate, it is getting me down.

OSCAR: Sorry to hear this Adam, yes this can be a side effect of the medication. Tell me a little bit more about what you are experiencing with the side effects? What ideas have you had about what you would like to be done? We can see what is realistic before your psychiatrist appointment.

In Box 7.3, Oscar acknowledges that Adam is struggling. This is sometimes called 'validation' in counselling and psychotherapy. He also requests more information from Adam using the phrase 'tell me', so Adam is invited to give more information and really air his concerns. Adam will notice that he is being listened to in this scenario; he now has some power and choice in what the next step might be.

The funnel of communication

The difference between the first and second scenarios in Boxes 7.2 and 7.3 is essentially the use of the 'tell me' request and the 'what' question, which is an 'open' question. It allows Adam to tell Oscar what is on his mind and share his ideas. When we interact with patients, there are times when we need to offer opportunities for them to air their own ideas about the way forward. Many people working in health and social care feel that, if they provide the patient with too much choice and decision making, the patient will be overwhelmed. There is no strong evidence for this, and it can be fear on the worker's part. It is how we communicate with the patient that is key. By asking Adam, 'What ideas do you have?', the support worker gets to listen to some possible solutions. Patients and clients often hold the answers.

> **Box 7.4 Scenario: Adam's reply**
>
> 'Yes, I have a couple of ideas, I don't know how realistic they are though. Do you think the psychiatrist could see me earlier? I know you won't be free to take me, but I have a friend who will go with me. My other idea is that I simply reduce the medication now as these are clearly side effects. Would this be possible?'

A helpful way of thinking about how we gather important information from patients and family can involve paying attention to how we, as practitioners, ask for information. Richards and Whyte's (2011) funnel of communication, shown in Figure 7.1, can be a helpful model to carry around in our minds when we plan conversations with patients and their families. If we require a rich amount of information, it is better to think about the wider parts of the funnel, and if we want to be more focused, with questions that require a simple yes or no, we can ask closed questions.

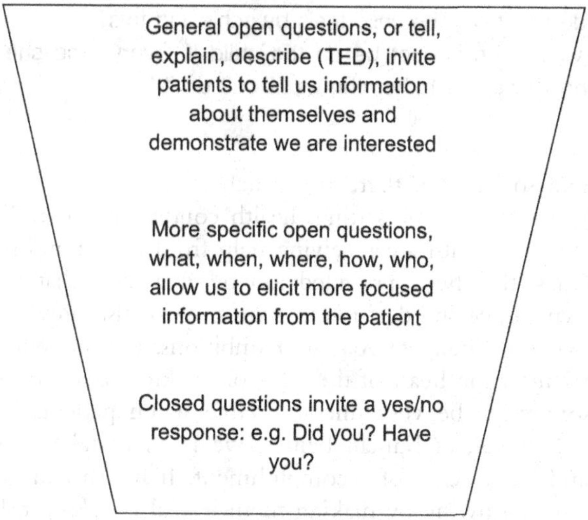

General open questions, or tell,
explain, describe (TED), invite
patients to tell us information
about themselves and
demonstrate we are interested

More specific open questions,
what, when, where, how, who,
allow us to elicit more focused
information from the patient

Closed questions invite a yes/no
response: e.g. Did you? Have
you?

Figure 7.1 The funnel of communication
Source: Adapted from Richards and Whyte (2011)

Box 7.5 Activity: Familiarise yourself with the funnel of communication

- Notice the impact of the use of open questions in the conversations you have at home or at work.
- Notice the impact of the use of closed questions in the conversations you have.
- Reflect on whether the person feels more listened to when responding to open or closed questions.

Positive risk taking

Positive risk taking is a healthy part of human behaviour. Children engage in it a lot while parents look fearfully on; see the example in Box 7.6. It is also a necessary ingredient if you are going to empower the people you work with to make independent decisions.

Box 7.6 Example: Child on a climbing frame

A 7-year-old child walks along the top of a climbing frame, jumps off the other end and beams from ear to ear at her father, who is watching and can finally breathe again.

- What do you think the child feels by achieving this?
- What would the impact be on the child if, every time she gets on a climbing frame, her father shouts, 'Don't do it!'

In health and social care, there is a much-documented concept called the 'sick role'. Depending on the setting, health condition, age and other factors, the people you work with are receiving help from health and social care services. Sometimes, the 'help' provided can be at a level that impacts on the individual's own choice and decision making and can also prevent people being able to fulfil some of their life goals and ambitions. Person-centred care wants to put the patient at the heart of the decision making, but services and practitioners can sometimes be very uncomfortable when patients take risks with their health. However, as human beings, we need to take risks in order to learn, grow and feel a sense of accomplishment. If health and social care prevents people from growing by making them fearful of taking risks, then there can be negative outcomes for patients in their lives but also in their engagement with the services providing support. The 'sick role' can occur, and this means that the person you work with starts to identify more as a patient needing help than as a person who has a life but just happens to need health input.

In your role as a support worker, patients might express their wishes and desires for the future. It is important to know that reaching our own personal goals in life can also be health enhancing. However, some goals that people want to achieve might also not be beneficial for the health condition they have been treated for. If you think about things in your own life that people have cautioned you against, it might be easier to put yourself in someone's shoes.

As a support worker, you might find yourself having the most contact with patients on a week-to-week basis and so you can often find yourself to be the link between the patient and the professional team. When patients open up and tell us their dreams and ambitions, it is a privilege and should be handled sensitively, as the response provided can cause damage to a patient's self-esteem and limit their view of the future. Positive risk taking should be encouraged, but it should not rest on your shoulders to agree that the patient can go ahead.

Box 7.7 Example: Positive risks

Siobhan, 21, is a wheelchair user. She has accepted a place at university. She has always relied on her mum for care and support. She wants to fully engage in student life, but her mum is apprehensive and is asking your advice about the risks involved. You are Siobhan's support worker and have known the family for 3 years.

How would you approach this with Siobhan and her mother?

Supporting difficult choices

The support worker may be present at the most difficult moments in a service user's and their family's journey through the health and social care system. You might be present when a family agrees with the medical team that their elderly loved one is no longer safe to go home. You could be there when a cancer patient is given the news that no other treatment is available and they have weeks to live. You might also be present when parents are told about a life-threatening operation that, if successful, could save the life of their child but, sadly, the odds are against it. These conversations might involve you directly or indirectly. You are not in a position of responsibility for the final decision making, but your opinion might count.

From person-centred to personalisation

Those of you who work with clients/patients with longer-term needs who require a range of service involvement might be familiar with the term 'personalisation'. Since the Labour government released a vision for adult social care, Putting People First (NHS 2007), there has been a focus on putting the client/patient at the centre of the decision making on their support needs. Earlier, we discussed the word 'empower'; the personalisation of care and support needs is based on the idea that the client is unique and does not always fit neatly into the traditional services available; therefore, they should be able to pick and choose.

According to the NHS Long-term Plan (2019), by 2023–2024, 200,000 people will benefit from what is called a personal health budget (PHB). The PHB is not a new entitlement for the patient, but a way of personalising funds for care and support based on the person's health and well-being needs. You might already, therefore, be working with clients because they have long-term needs and have chosen to fund your services using the process of direct payment. Their needs have been assessed by their local councils. This puts the client at the heart of the financial decision making as well as the care decisions. People can also select services you provide because of something they feel fits with their health and social care needs, or you could be working within an organisation that fits their cultural and social needs.

Privacy and dignity

We are all patients at some point in our life and have a medical or health/social care professional enquiring about personal aspects of our life. At the moment we request help, we relinquish some control and hand over to a stranger who we must trust will be able to respect the parts of us, both physical and psychological, that we would usually hide from those around us. The reason we hide these parts of ourselves or reveal them only to loved ones can be informed by culture, faith-based practices, sexuality, societal taboos or many other reasons that you could add to the list. Being prodded, poked or intimately examined by a professional stranger usually causes anxiety to most of us. We can have some very difficult thoughts that will make us behave in ways that are challenging to those around us. For practitioners, it can be easier to focus on the task at hand – for example, washing – rather than the person.

Box 7.8 Example: Mrs Jones

Mrs Jones (77) is being taught by you to transfer from her bed on to the commode in her home. You have met twice. She keeps asking you whether you are qualified to do this and quite often takes a swipe at you with her hand.

- What do you think she might be thinking?
- What do you think you can do to demonstrate you are working to respect her dignity and privacy where possible?

Confidentiality and social media

You are expected to adhere to your organisation's policies that inform employees how to manage confidential information and data. It is important, therefore, that you uphold this practice outside your work. You could be charged with gross misconduct if you breach confidentiality or reveal the identity of the people you work with. Today, most of us will carry a smartphone and make use of social media, perhaps to express our thoughts and opinions or share images of our lives as we go through our day. To uphold the dignity and privacy of service users, your colleagues and the organisation you work for, think about what you post before you post it. If your organisation has a policy for use of social media, please ensure you read it carefully. Box 7.9 has some questions to ask yourself before you post, as it could end your career in the field if you act unwisely.

Box 7.9 Questions

- Will the post breach the confidentiality of the people I work with?
- Will the post put vulnerable people I work with at risk?
- Will the post violate the dignity and respect of people I work with?
- Will the post bring my organisation into disrepute?
- Will the post cause damage to my colleague's reputation?
- Will my current employer or future employers act against me as a result of my post?

Safeguarding

Living without exposure to harm and abuse is a basic human right, but the sad evidence is that some of us are more vulnerable to the risk in our society than others. Safeguarding is a set of measures to ensure that all of us, but especially vulnerable adults, children and young people, are protected from abuse, harm and neglect in society. Organisations you work for have a duty to act to protect the safety and welfare of children and vulnerable adults. We have seen from examples in earlier chapters where things have gone badly wrong for these groups, and, sadly, examples continue to emerge year on year. The care sector does not always attract compassionate human beings, and, as workers, we must be watchful and know what to do if we have concerns. You, too, have a responsibility not to cause harm.

'Always make sure that your actions or omissions do not harm an individual's health or wellbeing. You must never abuse, neglect, harm or exploit those who use health and care services, their carers or your colleagues' (Skills for Care and Skills for Health, 2013, p. 5).

Safeguarding and your responsibilities

The organisations you work with will have a safeguarding policy. Please finish this section by having a look at it.

Box 7.10 Steps to take if a person is at risk

What steps should you take if you fear a person is at risk?

- Alert your line manager/supervisor and take advice
- Follow policy and procedure detailed
- Record actions and decisions
- Alert emergency services – fire, police, ambulance
- Communicate and respond to those professionals – for example, social services – whose duty it is to formally assess the risk and respond.

Children and young people

In society, it is understood that children and young people are a vulnerable group that the adult world can take advantage of, exploit, abuse and do harm to. It is everyone's business to protect the welfare of all children. Health and social care and education work with and, therefore, have high levels of contact, either formally or informally, with children and young people who may be 'vulnerable' or at risk because of life circumstances or the adults who care for them. If you are in contact with children in a professional capacity, either directly providing a caring duty or working with those who care for them, you will have duty to act when you fear a child is at risk from abuse, harm and neglect. The welfare of children in society is everyone's responsibility.

Vulnerable adults

Vulnerable adults include those people receiving care in their homes and people with sensory, physical or mental impairments. If you work in a care home, hospital or in the community, including for organisations that provide services but do not belong to the NHS, you will have a duty to safeguard those at risk of harm, too.

Abuse

The Care Act (2014) identifies ten types of abuse that, as a worker, you will need to be alert to (see Box 7.11). Please look into these further if you are not clear what they mean or seek guidance from your employer.

Box 7.11 Types of abuse

1   Physical abuse
2   Emotional/psychological abuse
3   Financial abuse
4   Sexual abuse
5   Organisational abuse
6   Neglect
7   Discriminatory abuse
8   Domestic violence
9   Modern slavery
10 Self-neglect.

Mental health awareness

One in four of us will experience a mental health problem over our lifetime, and so poor mental health is a very common experience (www.time-to-change.org.uk/about-mental-health). However, health and social care workers can still hold and reflect some stigmatising views about mental health problems. It has been a common myth that people with serious mental health problems are not capable of making decisions and shouldn't be allowed to take risks because they might be unpredictable. This has sometimes interfered with a support worker's ability to offer choice and opportunities for decision making, and, therefore, they are no longer 'person-centred' in their approach. The health and social care sectors have traditionally separated physical services from mental health services, although things are changing now. It has not been helpful to our patients to separate the body and the mind, as we are both.

Those of us with mental health problems will have good days and bad days. You will work with people who live with difficult thoughts, feelings and moods and might behave in a way we find unusual. You are not a psychiatrist, but you are still tasked with demonstrating the six Cs. The major mental health diagnoses, such as depression, anxiety and psychosis, are relatively common. At the more difficult end of the mental health spectrum, where things are very difficult, poor mental health can reduce an individual's capacity to take care of themselves, communicate and behave in a way that is easily understood, unless time is taken. It can be easy to start to take away their control and independence, but, actually, the role of the support worker might be to hold out the hope of recovery, offering respect and dignity when the other person hasn't got the resources.

Dementia

Dementia is a catch-all term for more than 200 brain disorders, according to Dementia UK (www.dementiauk.org), and is described as a syndrome for a collection of symptoms, the most recognised being memory loss, but there are many more. It is a common misconception that it is only the older person who is at risk: it is not a natural part of ageing disease at all. Most older people do not develop dementia (Jenkins, Ginesi, and Keenan 2016), and there are more than 40,000 people in the UK under 65 who have been diagnosed. You can have dementia alongside any other health condition, which means, in a caring relationship, you might be working with a person who has dementia but also, for example, diabetes or cancer.

It is recommended that you take opportunities (if you haven't already) for further training in dementia, as both a member of the public and a responsible professional. It can help dispel some of the myths about dementia only involving a person losing their memory. It can also support you to see 'the person' and understand how relationships are still important for this population of people who can still be strongly independent and have desires and wishes for the future, which can sometimes be difficult when communication and behaviour are challenging.

Conclusion

This chapter has focused on person-centred care and what that means to you as a support worker working with people who are vulnerable to being overlooked by a powerful health and social care sector that often tells them how to make choices and decisions. We hope you can see the importance of ensuring that, in your work with patients and service users, you offer conversations that are empowering and show the patient that you can see the whole person, beyond the caring needs they have.

References

Care Act (c 23). (2014). London, HMSO.

Health Foundation. (2016) Person-Centred Care Made Simple. www.health.org.uk/sites/default/files/PersonCentredCareMadeSimple.pdf (accessed 17 September 2020).

Jenkins, C., Ginesi, L., and Keenan, B. (2016). *Dementia care at a glance*. Chichester, UK: John Wiley.

Kenward, L., Whiffin, C., and Spalek, B. (2017). Feeling unsafe in the healthcare setting: Patients' perspectives. *British Journal of Nursing*, 26(3), 143–149.

NHS. (2007). Putting People First: A Shared Vision and Commitment to the Transformation of Adult Social Care. London: HM Government.

NHS. (2019). The NHS Long Term Plan. www.longtermplan.nhs.uk/publication/nhs-long-term-plan/ (accessed 30 June 2020).

Richards, D. and Whyte, R. (2011). *Reach out: National programme student materials to support the delivery of training for psychological wellbeing practitioners delivering low intensity interventions* (3rd edn). London: Rethink.

Ross, A. (2016). On learning from (being) the patient. *Psychodynamic Practice*, 22(3), 273–277.

Salomsé, G.M., Openheimer, D.G., Almeida, S.A., Bueno, M.L.G.B., Dutra, R.A.A., and Ferreira, L.M. (2013). Feelings of powerlessness in patients with venous leg ulcers. *Journal of Wound Care*, 22(11), 628–634.

Skills for Care and Skills for Health. (2013). Code of Conduct for Healthcare Support Workers and Adult Social Care Workers in England.

Recommended websites

www.alzheimers.org.uk

www.time-to-change.org.uk/

8 Know how to be competent in your current role

Paul Mackreth

Introduction

As you have identified from the previous chapters of this book, delivery of health and social care is fraught with difficulty and can be complex to understand, let alone to put into practice. Yet, when delivering care and support, we are often not aware of this as we often feel self-assured in what we are doing. But are we? How do we know what we are doing is safe?

Health and social care organisations often call our safe practice 'competence'. Systems and strategies are put in place to 'assure' competence. After all, any errors or omissions in our work can cause serious harm or even result in pain and death. So, knowing that we are competent in our role is an important aspect of our practice. Employers also carry liability for the quality of care.

Some textbooks aim to detail policy and procedures to guide you through doing things safely and well. We take a different approach in this chapter. We do not seek to tell you how to do something well, but guide you to consider the different aspects of competent practice, how you learn and where you can get help and where you can get support for your skills. A key aspect of this is being open and honest with yourself about your skills and continuously gaining feedback from those around you.

As educators in health and social care, we are often alarmed by students who say to us, 'I know how to do everything'. These are the scariest members of the health and social care team, as they do not acknowledge how practice can change or how we are all continually learning. They do not know their own limitations. We assert that, through being open to learning and being humble about new ideas, you can practise with competence.

This chapter is the culmination of many others in this handbook. It acts as a tool to ask you to 'assure' your own practice. It precedes the final chapter that can help you develop your career once you have consolidated your skills in your existing role.

Box 8.1 Activity: Recently completed tasks

Consider any task you have done recently:

- Where did you learn how to do it?
- When did you learn how to do it?
- If you did the task wrong, what harm could be caused?
- When did you last update this task?
- If you were challenged as to 'why' you did the task a certain way, could you explain?

Learning outcomes

At the end of this chapter you will be able to:

- Describe what support worker practice competence entails
- Detail the importance of practice competence and how you learn best
- Compare support worker competence with that of professional staff
- Articulate the boundaries of your own scope of competence.

Setting the scene

Knowing that we provide safe and effective care is a central tenet of any care system – doing good, while doing no harm. In the wider sphere, we all learn new things, practise them and then become proficient. However, in health and social care, our ability to learn by 'trial and error' is limited because of the harm it can cause. With very few courses or formal learning opportunities, health and social care workers are often 'apprenticed' in new roles – that is, they spend time on the job, training with a person with more experience or, if they are lucky, a trusted educator. You may have also spent time in a college or school. This learning would have culminated in an examination or observation of rights and wrongs.

To some extent, this is still how we learn. The current UK government (in 2020) is looking at reinvigorating apprenticeships as formal qualifications. However, for most support workers, their training has been less formal than this. Judgements as to safety and 'competence' are left to the individual to make or left to organisations to decide what support workers are 'allowed' or 'trained' to do by their own organisation. Interestingly, Griffin, Dunkley-Bent, Skewes and Linay (2010) carried out a study that found that maternity support workers were often trained 'in house', leading to a lot of role confusion given that some maternity support workers were highly skilled whereas others were more concerned with clerical or housekeeping duties. This led to a lot of confusion about boundaries of roles. We have found that support workers are often allowed to take on additional tasks when departments are busy, and then these tasks are withdrawn when it is not so busy!

In our own experience of running courses for support workers, we often find that workers can express to us what they should stop doing as much as they have learned how to do new things. What we detail below is a summary of what we think will help in your development and help you understand the background to learning so that you can deliver assured safe, effective and competent care for the best outcome for your clients.

Training and development

It is first worth considering how we learn; this additional understanding will allow us to consider what and how we learn best. Some books detail the work of Honey and Mumford (1986), who write about learner preferences:

- Activists learn through doing
- Reflectors observe and think
- Theorists read facts, concepts and models
- Pragmatists try things out.

Although models such as this are helpful in some situations, we prefer to review how and in what environment learning takes place. How we learn is a whole discipline of psychology, and so we can only touch upon it in this chapter and highlight how it relates to your role in support work.

Formal learning is a useful tool as it can set a baseline of things that people can learn. In a classroom, a tutor can direct what is right or wrong. Teaching is the emphasis where the tutor knows best and fills the students in the classroom with learning. It can be delivered en masse, and key messages are passed to students.

Many of us learned this way during our time at school. It is a helpful method when there are a lot of key facts that often remain unchanged – for example, in maths or basic science. We can also experience this method of learning through annual updates or in a conference setting on topics that interest us.

However, some may be put off by this style of learning. Some people do not respond well in a formal environment. You may lose concentration or become distracted. If you can't ask questions, the subject may be difficult to understand. As a result, we must consider that, just because there is a teacher 'teaching', it does not, therefore, mean that learning takes place! We also must trust that the teacher is skilled in keeping our attention, is interesting and is also correct in the knowledge that they are passing on!

It may be that the classroom does not and cannot replicate some of the challenges in our day-to-day practice. Despite these limitations, the ability to teach large groups and send consistent messages makes formalised learning in a classroom setting very popular.

It also allows learners to be assessed against criteria that can demonstrate that they are safe and have reached a minimum standard. You may have completed a care certificate that would be an example of this. We must stress that this only demonstrates that, at that time, you worked to this minimum standard. Practice changes over time, as does your approach to work; we sometimes cut corners or adapt what we do.

Learning from doing is an alternative or can support formal learning. It is based upon the well-known experiential learning cycle that Kolb (1984) based upon the work of another theorist called Dewey (cited by Ord 2012). Figure 8.1 shows a simple adaptation of the Kolb (1984) learning cycle, with support worker practice adaptations.

Learning from doing may appear obvious: just think about how you learned to ride a bike or to swim. However, in the context of care and support work, it is a method best known for learning from practice. This is not a 'passive' process, and it takes skill to 'reflectively learn' or to have 'reflective practice' – we detail how to do this in Chapter 2 of this book. As Chapter 2 articulates, reflection is a very active process. It allows us time to contemplate what we have done in practice and consider alternatives. We can build or scaffold our knowledge this way.

The problem people often find with reflection and experiential learning is that it takes a lot of skill and facilitation to do this. Professionally registered staff have a regulatory requirement to work in this way. The often cite mixed experiences of doing so, such as time to 'do reflection' and time to engage with alternative viewpoints through discussion or further reading.

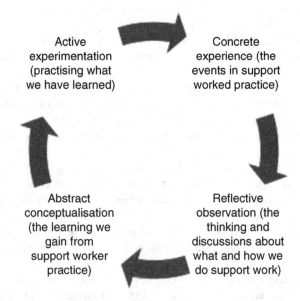

Figure 8.1 Learning cycle
Source: Adapted from Kolb 1984

Box 8.2 Activity: Example

Can you consider an example of where you have done this? It is probably easier to think of a negative example than a positive one, although we should also consider positive learning experiences.

To aid your thinking, we provide you with an example based upon Kolb's learning cycle:

- Concrete experience – knowing how to move someone with a hoist
- Reflective observation – all environments differ and sometimes cannot be adapted (e.g. furniture in a person's home)
- Conceptualisation – can we ask a person to move furniture?
- Active experimentation – asking a family to move furniture.

Theory and practice

We can build on 'learning through doing' by taking this experience and seeking what others have written about. This is when we reach being 'critically reflective' (Rolf and Freshwater 2010). There are some very well-known and very big challenges with this. Although it is logical to link best practice and theory to one's own practice, it is often described as 'the theory and practice gap'. It can take many years to put best evidence into practice; there is no one reason why, but we do know that dissemination of new knowledge is very difficult, and then changing practice is even more difficult again (Rogers 2003).

If you have time and access to a library, you can compare your practice experience with literature in the field of your practice. You can then make changes to your practice and encourage others to do so. This is the basis of most professional training courses such as nursing or occupational therapy. However, there are lots of different influences on your practice, such as custom, routine (Walsh and Ford 1989) and pressure to 'get on'.

Although this is a great aspiration, we do know that it is more probable that you will pick up best practice from other sources, such as practice guidelines, policy and procedures. What we would like you to learn is that reading and expanding what you know from books will always enhance your practice.

Development scales

Whatever the place and method of learning, it is important to note that we are never just suddenly able to know something new (Hayes and Mackreth 2008). We develop in areas of our practice over periods of time. It would be unfair to teach someone how to do something and then just expect them to do immediately; for this reason we don't like the term 'hit the ground running' that some people relate to when students/learners start to practice after formal programmes of learning – no one should be expected to learn something and then 'hit the ground running'. This crude expectation ignores that skills develop and are refined (and lost!) over time periods.

There are developmental scales to help us describe this process of 'development', two of them that we like are:-

1   Witnessed, Assimilated, Supervised and Proficient (WASP, Leeds Community Healthcare NHS Trust n.d).

   • Witnessed
   • Assimilated
   • Supervised
   • Proficient

2   Steinakre and Bell's (1979) experiential learning taxonomy:-

   • **Exposure** - (Observing something of interest, experiencing something that requires further investigation, researching and finding out more)
   • **Participation** - (Reviewing the situation, getting involved and exploring the wider picture)
   • **Identification** - (Processing the knowledge, recognising the need for change and development, interpreting the situation)
   • **Internalisation** - (Critical analysis and synthesis of the knowledge, adding personal ideas, improvement and transformation)
   • **Dissemination** - (Communicating transformation, sharing and spreading new ideas, sustaining developments)

Box 8.3 Activity: Scope to learn?

Consider something that you have learned recently, take each of these scales and consider at what stage you are at. Is there scope to learn more?

   • Witnessed
   • Assimilated
   • Supervised
   • Proficient

And:

   • Exposure
   • Participation
   • Identification
   • Internalisation
   • Dissemination

Competency debate

One thing is clear in practice: we should not do what we are *not* competent to do. Hayes and Mackreth (2008) found it helpful to clarify what a competency is and how it relates to competence; it is helpful to clarify this here:

- Competency: this is the descriptor of a role or function of a role.
- Competence: the measure, or lack, of a person's ability to undertake that role according to the description.

Understanding this brings up lots of questions, such as, who can assess competence? Is the competency written to an up-to-date standard? Does it reflect the full picture of what needs to be done to be safe?

These 'competency debates' are very long and detailed. Our own concern is with the full write-up of what needs to be included in a 'competency'. Undertaking a clinical task is a hugely complex area, and so to write it all down may get very 'task-orientated' and ignore the things that clients value most – the person-centred aspects of care and support. No one wants a robot looking after them.

A theorist called Bloom (1956, cited by Anderson and Krathwohl 2001) published a taxonomy (yes another one!) of learning indicating that learning has three main domains:

- Knowledge
- Skills
- Attitude.

The widespread adoption of competencies in our practice has allowed support workers to take on so much more in the clinical practice arena. As we have described in Chapter 3, this has opened up opportunities to develop new and exciting aspects of practice. But …!

Health and social care competencies are often referred to in terms of clinical skills. However, if we adopt the Bloom taxonomy, then we should also write them in terms beyond the psychomotor element (the 'skill' element of performing of the task) as they also need to take into account the background knowledge that you have (often for problem solving if something goes wrong) and the 'attitude' to the task.

We feel that developing the correct attitude is central to most areas covered in this handbook. We cannot express enough what we have learned through our own practice *and* what our service users have told us. The worker with the right attitude is valued far more by clients. Yet the attitude domain is very tiring to maintain. This is a real challenge in practice that is explored by many other authors who call it 'emotional labour' (e.g. Smith 2012).

If you think about the last time you had a blood test or an injection, it is not just the dexterity of the person using a needle and syringe or other equipment that matters. It is the knowledge of that person (order of blood bottles, drawing up the right amount of fluid etc.) and also their reassuring, helpful and informative attitude. You would not have liked it if it was taken in the wrong way or by a person who was rude to you or did not know how to deal with a problem.

Yet, often competency booklets just focus on the skill of the task. They miss the full, 'holistic' competence (McMullen et al. 2003) that is really needed. Or they are delivered with a tick box approach that doesn't give you the chance to fully develop that skill. We urge you to consider this when you next undertake competency training. There is a lot for us all to learn. Despite these issues, competencies in practice still provide us with a method of assuring safety in practice.

We feel that you should be exploring the current areas that are set out in the care certificate (Cavendish 2013) with the above understanding that it is not just about 'ticking boxes', but also about knowing and having the correct attitude to practice.

Box 8.4 Activity: Training to assure competence

Have you undertaken any of the following training courses to 'assure' yourself that you have a minimum level of competence in practice?

- Care certificate standards, including mandatory training:
  - Current examples include fluids and nutrition, basic life support, communication, equality and diversity, record keeping, confidentiality and accountability
- Knowing employer expectations and policy standards on:
  - Lone working
  - Health and safety
  - Moving and handling
  - First aid (physical and or mental health).

Now that we more fully understand what and why we have practice competence, we turn our attention to how we can measure it. This takes us back to the first activity: if we were challenged why we were doing something, could we answer?

How to measure support worker competence and evaluate quality care

In our day-to-day lives, we do things, we drive a car, we cook and prepare food and we support our friends and family. We do this intuitively and we rarely look back to see if we could have done this better, although some people do. We need to bring this change about in ourselves ('knowing yourself' – Chapter 2). People who allow themselves to continually learn new ways of doing things that they have always done are probably the inspiration to others.

We can measure our own competence through listening to others and accepting feedback. Some employers do this using formal methods (e.g. a competence booklet) or in less formal, yet structured, ways, such as in team meetings. The important thing is to seek feedback, accept feedback and to change as a result of feedback. Be humble in our approach to learning and listen to others, especially the clients and service users.

'Knowing' how to be competent through feedback can include the following:

- Managers' appraisals
- Service user feedback
- Supervision
- Team meetings and team handover
- Reflective practice (see Chapter 2).

Just as a reminder: any conversations about clients and client care need to be held in a private setting and away from listening ears so as to ensure we do not breach client confidentiality. Talking to your partner at home is *not* an option as this is a breach of your code of practice (Skills for Care and Skills for Health 2013; GIG Cymru/NHS Wales n.d.; NHS Scotland 2009; Northern Ireland Social Care Council n.d.) and can also break the law (Data Protection Act 2018)

How to record and keep evidence of competence

So, now that you have considered what you need to be competent in and then detailed how you like to learn (called your learning preferences), you need to turn your attention to how you detail and record your competence.

If you were born in the UK and went to school in the 1980s, you may recall you would have been given a brown faux leather file called your 'Record of achievement'. Every school leaver was provided with one to keep all of their certificates in. This could be described as a toast rack approach (Webb et al. 2002).

We now refer to these as 'portfolios' or 'profiles'. Casey and Egan (2010) wrote an article on how portfolios can be used and for what purpose. They indicate that profiles are different to portfolios and highlight the importance of portfolios in:

- *Being a vehicle for personal development* – you can detail your strengths and weaknesses so that you can highlight where you need to develop further
- *Adult learning* – they allow you the flexibility to learn as an adult learner; for example, they detail what you already have experienced and learned from

- *Professional profile* – they can include information relating to your work and self
- *Assuring quality* – they represent what you do
- *Detail prior learning* – so that you can evidence what you have learned formally or from experience
- *Evidence competence* – they demonstrate that you have the knowledge to be safe.

You will see that we are big advocates of keeping a portfolio because of the many different benefits that you can get from maintaining one. Inevitably though, we also know that you probably only look at putting one together when you are applying for a new job or a course. We advocate that you try to keep your portfolio up to date at all times and include in it your reflections upon practice. This can be in the form of a diary or logbook.

Conclusion

Overall, you need to ensure that what you do in practice is safe to do. If you don't feel comfortable, *stop* and take advice. Learning can be about what you should not be doing, as well as what you should be doing.

You need to assure yourself and other people that you are confident in your competence, and there are many ways that you can do this. You may want to match your own learning preferences to the forms of teaching that are available.

Competencies are important areas, but do consider whether these are 'gold standards' or minimum standards and also consider if they cover how you should conduct yourself in terms of attitude. It is only through doing this that you can truly become person-centred.

To ensure that you have done this and are up to date in practice, we advocate that you keep a professional portfolio of all of your work, your learning (both formal and informal) and courses that you have gained. This will help you in your career development, which is detailed in the next chapter.

References

Anderson, L.W. and Krathwohl, D.R. (2001). *A taxonomy for teaching, learning, and assessing: A revision of Bloom's taxonomy of educational objectives.* New York: Longman.

Casey, D., and Egan, D. (2010). The use of professional portfolios and profiles for career enhancement. *British Journal of Community Nursing*, 15(11), 547–552.

Cavendish, C. (2013). The Cavendish Review: An Independent Review into Healthcare Assistants and Support Workers in the NHS and Social Care Settings [Internet] www.gov.uk/government/uploads/system/uploads/attachment_data/file/212732/Cavendish_Review_ACCESSIBLE_-_FINAL_VERSION_16-7-13.pdf (accessed on 20 August 2013).

Data Protection Act (c 12). (2018). London: HMSO.

Griffin, R., Dunkley-Bent, J., Skewes, J., and Linay, D. (2010). Development of maternity support workers role in the UK. *British Journal of Midwifery*, 18(4), 243–246.

Hayes, S. and Mackreth, P. (2008). Methods of assessment. In: Smith, A., McAskill, H., and Jack, K. (Eds), *Developing advanced skills in practice teaching*. Basingstoke, UK: Palgrave, 94–107.

Honey, P. and Mumford, A. (1986). *The manual of learning styles*. Maidenhead, UK: Peter Honey.

Kolb, D. (1984). *Experiential learning: Experience as the source of learning and development*. Hemel Hempstead, UK: Prentice Hall.

Leeds Community Healthcare NHS Trust. (n.d.). Competency Portfolio for Non-Registered Staff. Unpublished.

McMullen, M., Endacott, R., Gray, M.A., Jasper, M., Miller, C.M., Scholes, J., and Webb, C. (2003). Portfolios and assessment of competence: A review of the literature. *Journal of Advanced Nursing*, 41(3), 283–294.

NHS Scotland. (2009). Code of Conduct for Healthcare Support Workers. The Scottish Government.

GIG Cymru/NHS Wales. (n.d.). Code of Conduct for Healthcare Support Workers in Wales. www.wales.nhs.uk/nhswalescodeofconductandcodeofpractice

Northern Ireland Social Care Council. (n.d.). Standards of Conduct and Practice for Social Care Workers. https://niscc.info/storage/resources/standards-of-conduct-and-practice-for-social-care-workers-2019-1.pdf

Ord, J. (2012). John Dewey and experiential learning: Developing the theory of youth work. *Youth and Policy*, 108, 55–72.

Rogers, E.M. (2003). *Diffusion of innovation* (5th edn). New York: Free Press.

Rolf, G. and Freshwater. (2010). *Critical reflection in practice: Generating knowledge for care*. Basingstoke, UK: Palgrave-Macmillan.

Skills for Care and Skills for Health. (2013). Code of Conduct for Healthcare Support Workers and Adult Social Care Workers in England. www.skillsforhealth.org.uk/standards/item/216-the-care-certificate

Smith, P. (2012). *The emotional labour of nursing revisited: Can nurses still care?* Basingstoke, UK, New York: Palgrave-Macmillan.

Steinaker, N.W. and Bell, M.R. (1979). *The experiential taxonomy: A new approach to teaching and learning*. London: Academic Press.

Walsh, M. and Ford, P. (1989). *Nursing rituals: Research and rational actions*. Oxford: Butterworth-Heinemann.

Webb, C., Endacott, R., Gray, M., Jasper, M., Miller, C., McMullan, M., and Scholes, J. (2002). Models of portfolios. *Medical Education*, 36, 897–898.

9 Know how to develop for new opportunities

Bryony Walker

Introduction

This chapter is designed to help you appreciate the importance of staying up to date in the health and social care field in which you work. It also wants you to consider your own career ambitions and how you might develop to go into other areas of the health and social care sector and appreciate potential for promotion within or beyond the field of support work.

Learning outcomes

At the end of this chapter you will be able to:

- Understand the importance of staying up to date
- Identify opportunities for further training/education
- Consider future career ambitions.

Setting the scene

Imagine going to your GP with a health problem and finding out your doctor hadn't had any additional training or continuing professional development since they qualified in 1990. You might question their ability to make an up-to-date diagnosis, and this would not inspire any confidence in their competence when you went for your appointment. Your concerns, as a patient, would be legitimate. Medicine is always changing for the better, with new advances in research that lead to new treatments, and so GPs need to update their training. There are also backward steps in medicine that GPs need to know about too, where treatments they have prescribed have had seriously adverse effects on the patient population and have had to be withdrawn. For example, in 2005, Thioridazine (Mellaril or Melleril), an antipsychotic drug widely used in the treatment of schizophrenia and psychosis, was withdrawn worldwide because it caused severe cardiac arrhythmias (heart irregularities) (Purhonen et al 2012).

Lifelong learning

In previous chapters, we have discussed self-awareness and professional development. However, in our experience of teaching many students in support roles and from support backgrounds, education, as in actively engaging in an academic course that results in assessment of knowledge and skills, might not be what you have considered to be your comfort zone. Depending on your age as you read the book, the evidence suggests that those in support worker roles come from a variety of educational backgrounds. Some of you will already have been to university and have degrees that might be related to health and social care, or you might have studied in another field entirely. You may have come to your role in health and social care via the further education (FE) route. Many of you may have left school at 16 and never even looked back at the school gates, and, lastly, some of you might have gained your qualification outside the United Kingdom. Educationally, you are a very mixed group of people, which is excellent news for your clients, as they are too.

Continuing professional development

As a support worker in health and social care, you do not (at the time this handbook was written) have a UK-wide, unified professional or regulatory body you belong to, unlike nurses, social workers and occupational therapists, whose professional bodies request their practitioners to evidence active engagement in CPD. For example, at the time of writing, every 3 years a registered nurse or nursing associate must revalidate their registration with the Nursing and Midwifery Council (NMC). However, as you can see from the following examples provided, the different codes of conducts or practice clearly mention ongoing development of knowledge and skills. Therefore, as a support worker, you should be supported by the organisations you work for, via your supervisor and/or line manager, to update your skills as much as possible.

Box 9.1 Codes of conduct/practice

England

> 6 Strive to improve the quality of healthcare, care and support through continuing professional development.
>
> (Skills for Care and Skills for Health 2013)

Wales

> 6 Improve the quality of care to service users by updating your knowledge, skills and experience through personal and professional development.
>
> (GIG Cymru/NHS Wales n.d.)

Box 9.2 Benefits of CPD activity to you and your clients

- Your clients may receive an improved caring experience
- Fewer complaints
- Education and training can build confidence to question practice that does not benefit the client
- Professionally and personally rewarding for you
- Your supervisor/manager might notice your motivation and dedication and provide you with more opportunities to develop or consider you for promotion.

Learning as adults

How we learn as adults differs from when we learned as children in school. In the early 1980s, an academic educator called Malcom Knowles generated five assumptions about adult learners. Look at the summarised and adapted list in Box 9.3 and try to apply the assumptions to yourself.

Box 9.3 Assumptions about adult learners

1   *Self-concept*: As we mature, we become more self-directed rather than dependent on others.
2   *Adult learner experience*: Maturity brings experience, which means lots of previous learning experience that can be useful to future learning experiences.
3   *Readiness to learn*: You will see the sense in learning if it has something to do with the roles you have in life.
4   *Orientation to learning*: As a person matures, their time perspective changes from one of postponed application of knowledge to immediacy of application, and, accordingly, their orientation towards learning shifts from one of subject-centredness to one of problem-centredness.
5   *Motivation to learn*: As we mature, the motivation to learn is internal. In other words, we do it because it is what we want to do or we understand it is important to do.

(Source: Adapted from Knowles 1984)

Learning technologies

If you are making a return to learning and education after a significant pause, you can expect that technology will be part of the learning process, and so some of the language might have changed. It is now possible to engage in learning remotely, as well as face to face. Virtual learning environments, or VLEs, are used to enable students to store their learning materials but also to enable students and teaching staff to interact via email or group task. You can also find that reading lists are available online, and some electronic reading resources are made available by tutors.

Education and Covid-19

Since the start of writing this book, the Covid-19 pandemic has changed the style of delivery of health and social care courses. At the time of writing, owing to the Covid pandemic, many students have been engaging in teaching and learning remotely, from home. Different platforms have been used to provide face-to-face remote learning, such as Zoom, Microsoft Teams and Skype. It is possible to have what is called a 'synchronous' lecture delivered in real time on these platforms and for students to be present from their workspaces in their home. It is possible to use these platforms for small group activities, too, and for students to be able to ask questions, discuss and chat about the topics they are learning about. This sudden and required shift to online learning might leave its mark, so that, in the future, students might find they are working from home using technology, rather than on campus.

How to stay up to date

Your employer and certainly the patients you work with are hoping you are dedicated and passionate about the role you fulfil and want you to be up to date and knowledgeable. The real-world experience is that training and education budgets in health and social care are subject to change, so that, although your employer agrees that, in theory, it would be marvellous for you to go to a conference in London on support worker roles in diabetes care, they may not agree to fund it owing to the limits of staff training budgets. It might be that you need to be very clear in your enthusiasm for professional development by requesting a formal meeting to discuss training and development opportunities with your supervisor or manager. NHS trusts and local authorities will have a training budget for staff and might need to meet targets for staff development. You can find a lot of training opportunities within larger organisations, which might be promoted via the intranet; however, the challenge is always to manage your diary and meet your work commitments. A healthy team approach will allow for people to cover other people's duties while a staff member is away on training, but obviously this can mean planning ahead.

Career progression

As a support worker/care worker or however your role is defined within your organisation, you are a key member of the workforce; we hope this book is giving you this message. However, you may wish to progress into one of the professional roles that exist within health and social care. There are various options available to you, but it is advisable that you take some preparatory steps before you make the decision.

Regulatory and professional bodies

If you are in a conventional health and social care setting, you may have heard your professional colleagues mention their regulatory bodies and professional bodies. Many of the professions in health and social care have 'protected titles', and, once qualified, a professional must register with them. The regulatory and professional bodies provide each qualified professional with a registration number, and it is, therefore, possible for a member of the public to check they are being treated by a qualified professional. Interestingly, 'nurse' and 'doctor' are not protected titles on their own: the protected title is 'doctor of medicine' and 'registered nurse'.

Box 9.4 Professional and regulatory bodies

The Health and Care Professions Council (HCPC; www.hcpc-uk.org/) is a regulatory body setting the standards for the following professions at the time of writing:

- Dietician
- Occupational therapist
- Physiotherapist
- Speech and language therapist
- Radiographer.

The NMC (www.nmc.org.uk/) performs the same regulatory responsibilities for nurses and midwives and, since 2018, nursing associates. For your information, if you are currently working as a healthcare assistant in the NHS, at the time of writing this book, the RCN had this statement on its website: 'The RCN supports mandatory regulation of HCAs and APs' (www.rcn.org.uk/professional-development/uk-wide-information-for-hcas-and-aps).

The General Medical Council (GMC; www.gmc-uk.org/) is the registration body for all doctors.

Social Work England (www.socialworkengland.org.uk/) is the registering body for social workers in England.

Social Work Scotland is the professional body for social workers in Scotland (https://socialworkscotland.org/about-us/).

Gofal Cymdeithasol Cymru (Social Care Wales; https://socialcare.wales/) maintains the register for social care and domiciliary workers in Wales. To be on the register, social care workers must demonstrate that they fulfil specific criteria including following a code of conduct. As a registered social care worker, you will be expected to engage in ongoing learning and development and maintain standards and competency befitting your role and duties.

Apprenticeships

In 2017, the government introduced the Apprenticeship Levy, which is an England-only tax on English employers with an annual wages bill of more than £3 million. In England, if you work for an employer that falls under the levy, you may have the opportunity to be released to study, for example, for a nursing degree apprenticeship; you will be paid by your employer, and the length of the course might be different to a full-time course as you are working rather than on an undergraduate programme. A new role has also recently been added to the nursing field called nursing associate, which is designed to 'bridge the gap between health and care assistants and registered nurses' (RCN 2018). There also apprenticeships opportunities here.

Shadowing

If your intention is to move forward in your career to train and qualify in one of the professions, it is really recommended and advisable to spend some time talking to or observing, if appropriate, members of that profession in action in the field. For example, if you wish to qualify as a nurse and work with the elderly, think about how you might make contact with a nurse working in the area. Prepare in advance for the meeting so that you can ask them important questions.

Box 9.5 Suggested questions

- Do you enjoy your work?
- What are the responsibilities and duties you have?
- What are your shift patterns?
- What are the challenges you face in your work?
- How do manage your work–life balance?
- Do you get a lot of opportunities for further training?

Qualifications

Courses in health, social care and medicine are mostly found in the sector of higher education (HE), although there can be some exceptions. To qualify as a nurse, occupational therapist, physiotherapist, social worker, speech and language therapist or dietitian, you will need to get a degree, which usually takes 3 years full time to complete. If you already hold a degree, you can find some master's programmes, but you will also need to meet the rest of the entry criteria, which usually include English and Maths GCSCEs. You will need to meet the entry criteria for the course you are interested in. It is wise to spend some time looking at courses. It is also possible to call and chat to someone, perhaps the course leader.

For entry on to professional courses such as nursing, social work or occupational therapy, you need both GCSCEs and A levels or A level equivalents. The University and Colleges Admissions Service (UCAS) website (www.ucas. com/) is a good place to start your research to identify how you meet the entry criteria. If you already meet the entry criteria, you can apply to your chosen institution via UCAS.

Foundation degrees

A foundation degree is a 1- or 2-year course before entry on to a full degree course. You can find various opportunities to study in both FE and HE. The entry criteria will vary from institution to institution, but these awards have been designed to support students to gain access to a degree pathway. They are also increasingly being made available to students who would not consider themselves to be the 'right' kind of person to consider a degree.

A new post

If you would like a change from your current role, the next question is where to look for opportunities. If you want to stay within your organisation, and these days employers would prefer staff stayed, make sure you check the intranet for opportunities. However, you may wish to change employer for many reasons, and there are a lot of places to look online or maybe via word of mouth. In recent times, large employers themselves have been known to host events for recruitment purposes, so please look out.

Applying for a new position

Depending on the employer, you will have a written application process to go through and also an interview. In preparing to apply, please do ensure you read all the job specifications and, in your application, ensure that you can meet all the essential requirements the employer asks of you. If you can demonstrate the desired qualities, this is even better. Those applicants who do not address essential requirements will be very low down the list to reach the next stage of the application process and can expect to be disappointed.

Temporary/hourly paid work

For many reasons, such as family or caring responsibilities, you might not wish or be able to commit to a full-time permanent position but require more flexibility in your work role. You might also want to get experience across a range of care areas. At the time of writing, there are many opportunities in health and social care to work this way. You can easily search on the internet, of course. You will find recruitment agencies and care agencies but might also find that organisations keen to recruit host their own recruitment events.

Just a word of caution about temporary work or working for a care agency as 'peripatetic' staff. Peripatetic means the work can change from one care setting to another with great frequency, and so there can be a different skills mix required. The agency will expect you to be flexible and adaptable to the environment. The phrase 'hit the ground running' is sometimes used here. You will need to find out from whomever is in charge what is expected of your role and be transparent about your own limits of understanding about the setting you find yourself in and/or training, so that patients are not put at risk. You will need to be happy to ask questions of staff around you who might not really consider you to be a part of the team.

Current and previous employer references

It is standard practice to request references in the workplace. However, you will be working with vulnerable people, and so the prospective employer needs to be extra vigilant in order to be satisfied you will be a practitioner who will be safe, and they will follow up on references for this reason and ask questions about your ability to work with integrity. You need to think about who will represent you truthfully in a reference. If you have a supervisor or line manager who can vouch for your integrity in the workplace, this is the best person to ask. If you are in a position to apply for a position but are new to the field of health and social care, you might request a reference from a previous employer, even if you were in a volunteer position. Educators who have perhaps taught you in the field of health and social care are also people to approach. Please do not forget that you can call the organisation and ask; this does show you are interested in the post and prepared to problem solve.

DBS checks

A DBS (https://dbscheckonline.org.uk/) check will be carried out by employers and educational institutions that offer placements to check whether or not you have a criminal record. There are different levels of check (basic, standard and enhanced) available, according to the level of vulnerability you are working with. The enhanced DBS is for vulnerable adults and children.

The interview

How to prepare

If you have read the whole of this book, you should have taken the steps required of a self-aware practitioner who has a foundational knowledge and understanding of the complexities that you face being in a support worker role. You are now a reflective practitioner and you can use this self-knowledge and understanding to prepare for an interview.

Writing the application form

The application form will include a job description that will outline the role and duties of the job and will also include a list of requirements that an applicant needs to fulfil to be considered for the job. The forms will vary from service to service and will also be different if you are applying for a permanent position or if you want to work for an agency. Most applications will expect you now to have computer skills so that you can complete and submit online, but there may be a few that will send you a hard copy in the post. Please be aware that those tasked with short-listing (usually a representative from human resources and staff in management or senior practice positions) will be looking for an application that meets all the requirements for the position.

However, if you are reading this book and are working in a different sector – for example, retail or catering – there are a lot of transferable skills, especially if you think about skills such as working in a team and effective communication.

Managing nerves

You may be someone who handles interviews well and perhaps even enjoys the opportunity to showcase your experience and skills to those who interview you. It is unfashionable to say so, but there is nothing wrong with positively engaging with the prospect of being interviewed. Enjoying the experience might sound a strange idea, but interviews are fantastic learning opportunities. We do need to approach them realistically, however, as we cannot control the thoughts and minds of those who interview us. Most of us, at some point or other, will face disappointment, and the reasons for this can be countless.

For many of us, an interview can make us feel out of our comfort zone, and some of this might be linked to how we view ourselves and what we say to ourselves. If you approach an interview with an 'I probably won't get it' attitude, that does prepare you for failure, which can be oddly comforting, but it also does not allow you to explore the possibility of success, which can be scary. Exploring the possibility of success, however, allows you to focus on the goal of 'getting the job' and will help you take the steps to do so. Unfortunately, there is no avoiding the fact that other people may also be lined up to want the position as much as yourself, which can add an additional pressure. However, once you have been invited to interview, you are on an equal footing with everyone who is attending for interview. You have got through the first hurdle and should give yourself a pat on the back. As the day of the interview approaches, it is wise to revisit the job specification and see again exactly what the employers want to see in the person who will be successful in being offered the position. It is possible sometimes that an employer will set you a task so that they can see some of your skills and knowledge distilled into an activity, such as a presentation.

On the day, remember to dress in a way you feel comfortable but employable. In the interview, communicate your genuine enthusiasm for the role and be clear that you will be hardworking and happy to learn.

Box 9.6 Example of an interview question

Provide us with an example of good communication and when communication went wrong in your practice.

You will probably have provided examples in your written application about how effective you are at communication. In an interview, the panel will be observing your communication skills in action, as you go through the interview, as well as how you respond to questions. If you look at the above question, it is also really asking about your *self-awareness*, your *professional integrity* to be able to be *honest* about both the good and difficult experiences you have had in your practice.

Promotion

It is reasonable to hope that, as you gain experience in your chosen area of support work and demonstrate an active commitment to staying up to date, this should advance your prospects to gain promotion, and an all-important pay rise should be a possibility. In support work, as in the other job roles, you might have to look around for these opportunities, of course, but they are there. In earlier chapters, we have discussed how the role of support worker is a very broad umbrella term; however, the skills of self-awareness, ability to build relationships with vulnerable people and working in teams connect them all, and these are highly transferable skills that are relevant to many industries. Promotion can come in various forms; obviously, a new career path to qualify as a professional will take you on to a different pay scale. However, these days, health and social care delivery comes in many forms: within the NHS, social services, private business and charities. All these service providers employ significant numbers of support worker staff who need support, training, line management and leadership. Each organisation will make its own decisions about how the path to promotion looks. It might be wise to ask this question at interview.

The titles of these promotional positions can vary according to the sector. You might be in a large organisation that uses its website to advertise, so keep a close eye or, again, use some of the job websites used for health and social care positions.

Box 9.7 Examples of some promotion titles

- Team leader
- Senior care assistant
- Senior support worker
- Team manager

Assertiveness

If you want to be promoted or be considered for other opportunities, just be aware your organisation cannot mind-read, so it is you who will have to let them know your ambitions and intention to progress. You will, therefore, need to be assertive to let your line manager, supervisor or manager of service know. How you do this usually requires a clear and direct communication rather than one that hints gently with the expectation that you will be offered the opportunity. Care services are busy, high-demand environments where managers often feel like they are fire-fighting and so might not be in the zone to understand their staff's career intentions.

Mentoring and coaching

As you become more experienced in your field of practice, you may wish to take on additional responsibilities that focus on building the knowledge and competency of new staff. You might offer some mentoring or coaching to members of the team, in order to orientate them to the policies and practice of the service and how to work with clients and service users. Mentoring and coaching training is available as a qualification from organisations, and many organisations contract an external provider to deliver this, so it might be worth looking out for, or you might have a particular 'in house' programme that is delivered, or you might simply be asked to do this as an experienced member of the team. Mentoring and coaching of staff can be viewed by employers as a development opportunity, and so might not directly lead to promotion but can demonstrate to managers that you are keen to contribute.

Management and leadership

You might want to stay within the health and social care sector but reach a point in your career when you become more interested in the administration and organisation of services that impact on your clients' experiences of care. Traditionally, in health and social care, management and leadership roles can take you away from the hours of face-to-face contact with patients and clients, so do consider this before applying. Roles in management and leadership can also mean higher pay scales, as these roles are considered to require more complex skills and often are organisation-focused rather than working directly with the target population your service is offering care to.

Business and enterprise

There are also opportunities for business and enterprise skills in the health and social care sector. Indeed, some of the language of business might already come into your role as a support worker. You might be involved in audits, be aware of tendering processes and gather outcome information. At the time of writing, the sector is made up of service providers from the private, public and charitable sectors, but there are also gaps in provision identified by commissioners.

Conclusion

The purpose of this chapter has been to convey the importance of keeping up to date in the area you work in as a support worker, and that continuing professional development can have a direct impact on the quality of care you provide, but, also, investing in CPD demonstrates that your skills are valuable. We hope you will consider your future in the profession to be fulfilling and rewarding, but also that the field of health and social care can provide you with opportunities to fulfil career ambitions.

References

GIG Cymru/NHS Wales. (n.d.). Code of Conduct for Healthcare Support Workers in Wales. www.wales.nhs.uk/nhswalescodeofconductandcodeofpractice

Purhonen, M., Koponen, H., Tiihonen, J., and Tanskane, A. (2012). Outcome of patients after market withdrawal of thioridazine: A retrospective analysis in a nationwide cohort. *Pharmacoepidemiology and Drug Safety*, 21, 1227–1231.

Knowles, M. S. (1984). *Andragogy in action*. San Francisco: Jossey-Bass.

Royal College of Nursing. (2020). Becoming a Nursing Associate. www.rcn.org.uk/professional-development/become-a-nursing-associate (accessed 17 September 2020).

Skills for Care and Skills for Health. (2013). Code of Conduct for Healthcare Support Workers and Adult Social Care Workers in England. www.skillsforhealth.org.uk/standards/item/216-the-care-certificate

Index

Page references in *italics* indicate a figure; page references in **bold** indicate a table.

Printed in the United States
By Bookmasters